THE ROB LIPSETT
GAME PLAN

PENGUIN LIFE

UK | USA | Canada | Ireland | Australia
India | New Zealand | South Africa

Penguin Life is part of the Penguin Random House group of companies
whose addresses can be found at global.penguinrandomhouse.com.

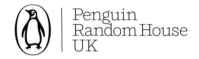
Penguin
Random House
UK

First published 2019
001

Designed by Nic&Lou
Colour reproduction by Altaimage Ltd
Printed and bound in China

A CIP catalogue record for this book is available from the British Library

ISBN: 978–0–241–35293–9

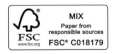

MIX
Paper from
responsible sources
FSC® C018179

greenpenguin.co.uk

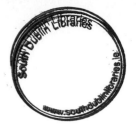

THE ROB LIPSETT
GAME PLAN

PENGUIN LIFE

AN IMPRINT OF

PENGUIN BOOKS

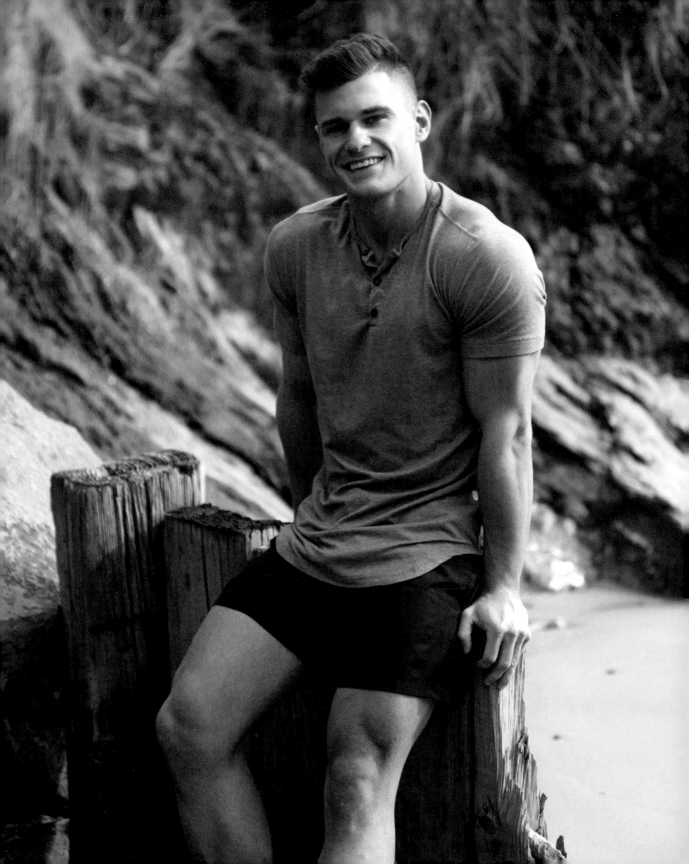

CONTENTS

What's going on, everyone?! Before we get down to business I want to thank you for picking up this book. It's the first step in what I hope will be a rewarding interaction between the two of us. Whether it's information, motivation or simply inspiration you gain, if you come away from reading this happier with yourself and with clear fitness and lifestyle goals identified, then my job here is done.

So let me start with a bit of background in what I'm all about.

My name is Rob Lipsett. I'm 26 years old and was born and raised in Dublin, Ireland. When I am asked to describe myself, I sometimes find it hard to put it into words or say what it is I do — the truth is I don't do just one thing!

- I'm an online fitness entrepreneur.
- I'm the owner of several businesses.
- I'm a YouTuber.
- I'm a qualified personal trainer.
- I'm an Instagrammer. (I like to make up my own words sometimes.)
- I'm a world traveller, investor, content creator and an author (as of now).

In other words, I do bits of lots of things, and sometimes when I'm not bothered to list all that I do I just tell people that I'm a guy who does stuff on the internet.

From that list it may sound like I lead a fun and exciting life, and it's true, I do, but I wasn't handed any of this and I didn't always love what I do. I didn't always wake up motivated to crush the day. In fact, I used to dread waking up.

I'm going to start at the beginning, when things weren't so great. A place where you might be right now.

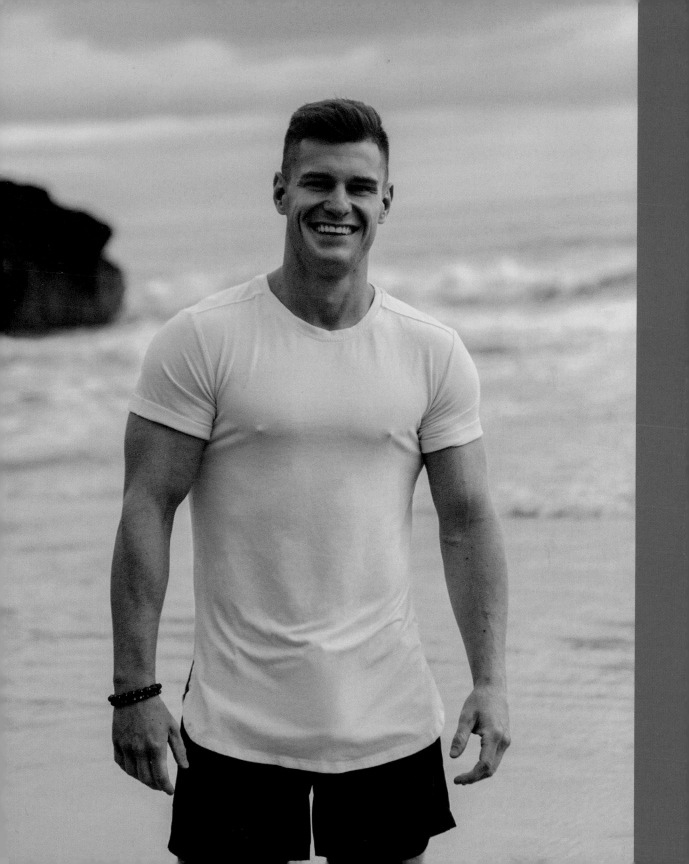

At 17, I was in an all-boys' secondary school. I was having a great time, but in every area except academics. I loved the sports, I loved the banter with the lads, I even loved the food. It was here that I discovered my passion for strength, fitness and training. I picked up a rugby ball at 12 years old and was always decent, but nothing spectacular. My real strength lay on the fitness side of things – running suicide drills, flipping tyres, morning weights before class and conditioning out on 'the farm' (basically a muddy field where we would lift heavy things). I loved it. I think it was because I've always been an uncomplicated guy – if you tell me to run from A to B, I'll do it, no problem, and do it well.

Despite all the training in the fields, hoovering up the nosh in the canteen and the craic with my mates, I wasn't doing great academically, especially in anything to do with maths or numbers. (Ironically, I now have no problem counting how many grams of protein I eat a day.) In June 2011, I sat my Leaving Cert and said goodbye to school. The Irish Leaving Certificate is a set of exams that earn you points, which in turn determine what course or college you get into. It's a bit like A levels in the UK, but with way more subjects. I did my best but wasn't expecting much.

When I went to pick up my results, I was so negative about the whole thing. Most students ripped open their letters straight away to see if they'd got into the course they signed up for, but I swear to God I didn't open mine for two days, as I wanted to go out that night and not be in a terrible mood and all mopey about my results. Pretty deadbeat and pessimistic, eh? I wasn't always the positive guy you see today. When I finally opened the envelope I found out I'd got into one of the business courses that I had applied for and decided to go along with it.

Seven years ago, Instagram was hardly a thing, I had never heard of vlogging and I thought the only way to make money on the internet was by being in X-rated movies. My mind was stuck in the groove that I had to follow the 'normal' path: go to college to do some course I was only mildly interested in, graduate, do an internship with low pay or no pay, get a job in a company, work under someone else to make someone else's company better even though it was highly unlikely that I would ever be at the top of said company, wait for the weekend to come and always know what day it was – 'Thursday, nearly there!' Then at the weekend go out to the same spots and get wasted, then feel terrible on Monday and do it all over again. For about 30 years. Deep down, I knew I couldn't do it.

> " I've always been an uncomplicated guy – if you tell me to run from A to B, I'll do it, no problem, and do it well."

> "The hidden potential that's waiting to be unlocked in so many people is actually mind-blowing."

I started my first year in college and it went similarly enough to school. Although the social life was epic and I was interested in business and stories about how people did amazing and exciting things in the world of commerce, I had very little motivation to work on the modules. They were still going on about Pythagoras' theorem for no good reason, and the marketing stuff was whack too. Even though I was still very young at this stage (about 20), I knew this wasn't going to help me get the life that I wanted. And looking back on it now, I was right.

I failed my first year of college, but my parents and year heads convinced me to repeat the year. I took their advice, and guess what? I failed the year again. I didn't blame them – they were from a different generation, so fair enough, they didn't know there were any other viable alternatives to that 'normal' path – but the hard reality was that I had stayed stagnant for two years in a row, with no progression, nothing new and nothing outstanding or memorable achieved. It really sucked, especially because our early twenties is a time of life when we're primed and ready to go, so full of energy and enthusiasm but often not in the right situation to utilize it. We're also led to believe that if we're not academic then we're stupid or slow-witted. When you get handed back multiple tests with a big fat F written on them, it's hard not to feel like you're shit at everything. But I wasn't – I just needed to find out what I was good at. And this applies to everybody, not just me. You could literally be the world's greatest at something and have no idea! How insane is that? The hidden potential that's waiting to be unlocked in so many people is actually mind-blowing.

So even though the whole college thing wasn't for me, I still think college can be great if you're studying a subject you're passionate about and that will have some relevance in the real world. The social aspect of it is important too. You'll learn a lot about yourself and get into some funny, character-building situations. Even though I did spend those two years in college spinning my wheels, I don't regret it. If I hadn't given college a go, I probably wouldn't be the person I am today. It's the butterfly effect in action – a theory that everything that has happened, even if it's something small, like a butterfly flapping its wings on the other side of the world, sets the circumstances in motion to make you into the person you are.

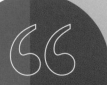

"If I hadn't given college a go, I probably wouldn't be the person I am today."

At this stage, I decided to start listening to myself. I sat on the side of my bed and took a long, hard look at my life.

- I was in my early twenties.
- I was not academic.
- I was not learning anything that I was passionate about in college.
- I was going between part-time jobs that were leading nowhere, and got fired regularly due to my lack of enthusiasm (I would have fired myself too, in fairness).
- I'd loved everything to do with training, nutrition and body composition since school. It was the only consistent thing in my entire life, the only thing I was really into.
- I loved socializing, going to new places and meeting new people.

So I said to myself, 'How can I make a living out of going to the gym, meeting people and having fun? That sounds like a complete joke! It's just not realistic. Get a grip, Rob. Life doesn't work that way. You can't just have fun and do what you love for a living.'

This was the turning point when I started to think differently.

I started asking myself 'Why not?' a lot. Whenever I doubted myself or thought, 'I can't do this', I would ask myself, 'Why not?' It was like those cartoons where you have a devil on one shoulder and an angel on the other. One was telling me 'You can't do this' and the other was asking 'Why not?' I'm glad I listened to the angel. I decided to drop out of college (which felt like a waste of time for me) and wing it to see what would happen.

Seeing as how I had no job and no college to go to, I had lots of spare time to not only hit the gym but to start working out my mind too. I devoured self-development books and listened to podcasts and interviews with people who were killing the game in their chosen fields. There was no single book I read or nugget of information I learned that changed me; it was an accumulation of constantly inhaling these positive guidelines combined with some common effing sense.

As I said earlier, I'm a really uncomplicated guy, which means I don't overthink things or go into a negative spiral when faced with a predicament. I'd say to myself, 'Look, it's cool. I'll sort this, I'll find a way around this. It could be worse, this isn't a big deal; there are actually some pros to this and lessons to be learned', etc. The negative way to react would be to freak out, worry, stress over it, list all the terrible things that will come from it, give up completely, complain, make excuses for yourself and blame others. Which option do you honestly think is the better one? When you say it out loud, it's obvious. Why would you ever act the other way? Why look at the glass as being half empty instead of half full? Not only is there no benefit to looking at life like that but it will only set you back and make matters worse.

I know it's easier said than done. I still have negative thoughts to this day and doubt myself at times, but I'm quick to snap out of it. I find it's extremely helpful to take a step back, apply some critical and logical thinking and literally ask myself out loud, 'Why think like this? What is the actual point of thinking negatively about this situation?' After a while, the positive outlook will become a habit that's encoded into your DNA. Trust me, you'll end up laughing at yourself for thinking those pointless negative thoughts. You'll give a proverbial middle finger to them and then shrug and 'LOL' to yourself.

Once I had exercised my brain and equipped myself with this new outlook on life, I decided to put it into action. There's no point listening to all the tips, tricks and advice in the world if you don't put them into action. My way of doing this was to follow through on my goals, dreams and passions in a concrete way. I loved fitness and I loved socializing, so posting my fitness endeavours and progress on social media was a bit of a no-brainer.

Instead of writing articles on a blog, I started writing informative fitness posts on Facebook and Instagram and dispelling common myths. Due to my massive interest in health and fitness from a young age, I had accumulated a lot of knowledge over the years (guess I wasn't so stupid after all!). People would tag their friends and say, 'Hey, did you know this? Check this out!' It got to the point where people would send me private messages looking for advice and training plans. I would critique their routines, answer any questions they had and even create new plans for free (humble beginnings).

> " There's no point listening to all the tips, tricks and advice in the world if you don't put them into action."

> **Posting my fitness endeavours and progress on social media was a bit of a no-brainer."**

I had a lot of fun doing this for a few months. For the first time in a long time I actually felt excited — genuinely excited — about something. Every time I clicked 'Share' on a post I'd get a rush of adrenaline. Eventually I got so many messages and had so many people asking about the same topics that I decided to make some videos on YouTube to answer those questions. Instead of writing out these long, individual responses every time, I could just link to one of my videos.

The videos went down well and got maybe 1,000 views to begin with. I had no money to invest in equipment and lighting — I had about €300 in my bank account from working in retail — but I was just happy to be talking about something I was actually interested in and to have a sense of fulfilment. I filmed all my first videos on an iPhone 5 and instead of using a tripod I just sellotaped the phone to a stack of cardboard boxes — half the time I couldn't even see if the video was still recording!

I still lived in the family home at this stage, and since I'm the youngest everyone else had moved out and all the rooms in my house were rented to strangers, like in a hostel or student accommodation, which isn't ideal when you're trying to become a YouTuber. My laptop and camera were routinely stolen from my room and people would walk into the kitchen when I was trying to record a 'professional' recipe video. But I didn't care. I just kept on producing content, writing posts on Facebook or Instagram and recording videos.

Then I started getting asked regularly for personalized plans or for ongoing support online, and that's when I had my light- bulb moment. The idea for my nascent business was staring me in the face, which is so often the case with business ideas. I simply came up with a solution to a problem that was being presented to me regularly. I went to a computing student I knew and asked him to make me a dead basic website that could take online payments. It cost me around €200 in cash and it crashed the odd time, but it was enough to get by on. So before going any further, let me tell you that yes, you can make a six-figure business out of a few hundred euro and a good work ethic.

We live in the most technological and entrepreneurial time in history. The planet is millions of years old and the internet has been around for 20-odd years – can you actually picture that timeline in your head? It's staggering how fast we are advancing and it has never been easier to get your message out there. If you have a good idea, then you literally have no excuses for people not to hear about your business.

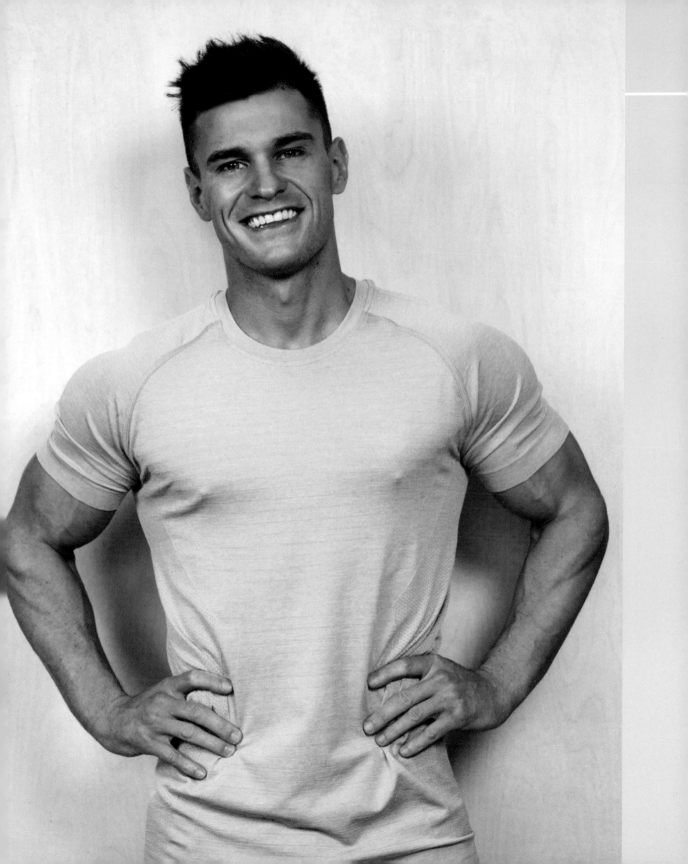

" I'm a big
believer that
small efforts
over time
can build into
life-changing
circumstances."

So that's how I started. Now multiply the above with more than three years of producing hundreds of hours of content, getting out into the world, putting myself in the right situations, investing everything I earned towards my goals, staying consistent and working my ass off. But it wasn't work to me. I was having the time of my life doing all of it. It's got to the stage where I'm literally sitting on a plane flying to an exotic location as I write these words.

I can't even express how grateful I am for all of this. I wanted to inspire other people to do the same and chase their dreams, which gave me the idea to start a company recently called The Creator Agency. The premise is simple: it's an events company that brings content creators together to positively impact the lives of others. So far we've held multiple events and the feedback has been nothing but amazing. There is nothing more fulfilling than having someone say you changed their life for the better — that's worth more than any amount of money.

I also recently participated in a TEDx Talk (TED-type talks that focus on local communities rather than global issues). The theme of the day was doing things that scare you, and some of the other speakers had gone through unimaginable adversity and struggles. Then there was me, some dropout who got fired from jobs and was too up himself to do what society told him to do. But I'll bet that there are a lot of people who are in a similar situation to where I was and could do with reading this.

I'm a big believer that small efforts over time can build into life-changing circumstances. I remember the first time I did a public speaking event. It was for a beauty bloggers' workshop and I was covering the health and fitness part of the day. I recorded it and watched it back and was really happy with it. I recently came across it on YouTube (four years later) and couldn't believe how far I've come. I used to say 'ehm' and 'uhm' every few seconds, my presence was weak, I had no flow, I sounded like I didn't fully believe in what I was saying, my voice was different and I wasn't nearly as confident as I am now. I struggled to speak for eight minutes. Now I host events where I speak and interview guests for five hours straight with only a ten-minute break.

When people ask me how I built up the confidence to do all this, I tell them to start making small improvements in the right direction, stay consistent and, most importantly, just start doing. I kept doing talks (often for free), kept making YouTube videos, kept networking and kept putting myself out there. I still do the same things to this day. I even began learning from other public speakers who put all their talks on YouTube. I quickly realized that it's not all about what you say, it's more about how you say it. If you're totally engrossed in what you're talking about, then it's likely that everybody else will be too. If you speak with conviction and talk about what you want to talk about, show leadership and know what you're doing, people will listen.

> "With each step forward, you become closer to where you want to be."

Never underestimate the small day-to-day efforts — they go hand in hand with taking massive action. With each step forward, you become closer to where you want to be. Over time, those small steps will add up to huge leaps.

This book aims to help you get the body you've always wanted while keeping a positive mindset and improving your health. My three-point action plan will help you to revolutionize your life for the better. First, we're going to address your fitness mindset to get your head in the right place to begin your new health and training regime. Then we'll work on nutrition, as it's so important to be eating well so that you can maximize your training. Then we're going to concentrate on training, where I've set out some great training plans that will get you into shape and tone your body in an achievable, realistic way. And finally, to top this all off, I've shared some of my favourite go-to recipes that are not only healthy but also taste amazing.

So what are we waiting for? Let's get started!

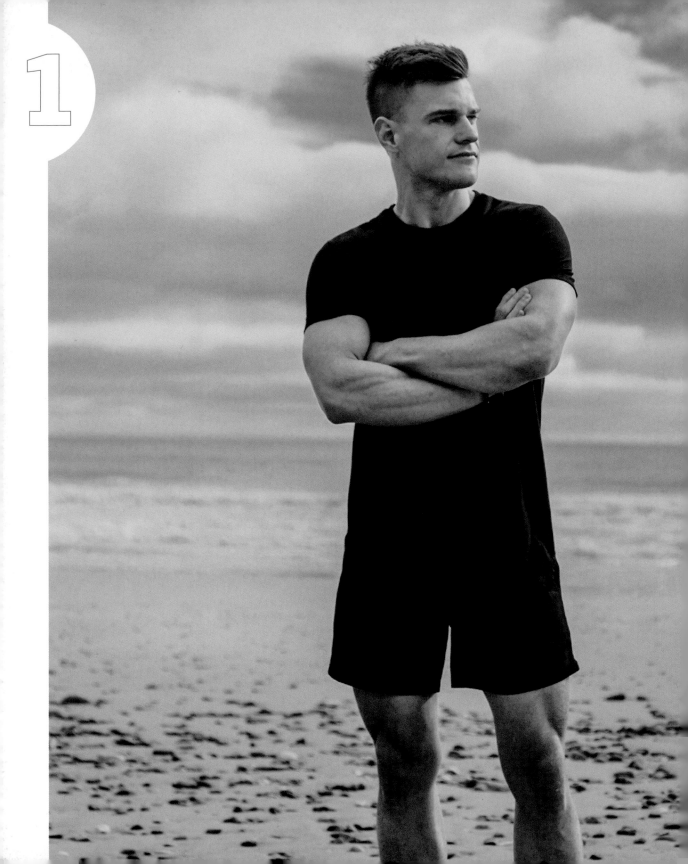

THE
MINDSET
PLAN

THE MINDSET PLAN

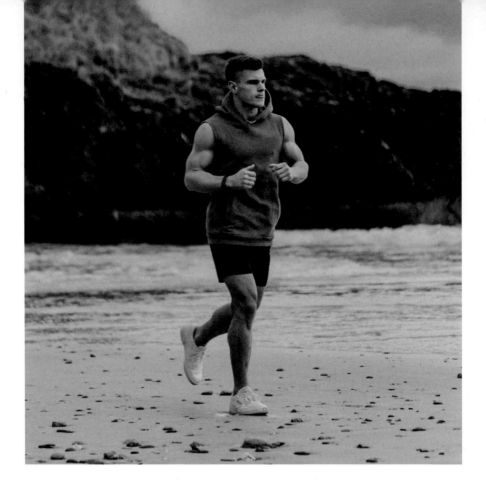

Before we get down to the nuts and bolts of getting lean and strong (for those, read nutrition and training), we first need to focus on a hugely important part of your body in your quest for great shape and fitness: your mind. In order to have your body in check, you've got to have your mind in check too or it will keep tripping you up — it's an incredibly powerful and persuasive voice! It will tell you things like, 'You're too old to start trying to get in shape now,' or 'You've been on this crazy programme for a month now and I don't see any results. It's tedious and tiring — just give up and go back to the sofa and box sets.' I'm going to hit you up with a few of my tried-and-tested principles and tips for getting your mind in check.

Mind in check = body in check ✓

Start small

If you're in bad shape and want to work towards having a healthy body that looks good and feels great, then you have to realize that you won't get there in a day. Time after time I see people fail to stick to a diet and exercise programme because they try to make too many changes at once and it all becomes too much and unsustainable. We're playing a long lifestyle game here, not a game of instant rewards. Baby steps are key when you're starting out. Set yourself small goals along the way — you'll feel rewarded for your efforts and the work you're putting in will be validated. Tell yourself:

- This week I'm going to run for 10 minutes more than last week.
- This week I'm going to lift heavier weights on my main compound lifts.
- This week I'm going to hold a longer plank.
- This week I'm going to plan some of my meals so that I don't end up reaching for unhealthy options because I'm too tired to cook after work.
- This week I'm going to be more conscious of my food choices and monitor my intake more accurately.
- This week I'm going to drink enough water.

"It can help to close your eyes and visualize yourself achieving your goal in, say, six months' time. Doesn't it feel good? Don't you look great?"

Cross those thresholds, feel good about it, then keep moving. Achieving your goals takes time, patience and hard work — it's a big help to be aware of that from the outset. There will be times when you'll feel as if you're going nowhere, when you want to quit because you don't feel like your efforts are being rewarded. In order to get through moments like these, you must also allow yourself to enjoy the process — you're getting fit and you're on the way, so allow yourself to feel a sense of accomplishment. It can help to close your eyes and visualize yourself achieving your goal in, say, six months' time. Doesn't it feel good? Don't you look great? The time will pass either way, so why not make the most of it?

Stop making excuses

It's so easy to tell yourself, 'Not today, I'll start tomorrow.' If you make excuses and go into something with that mindset, then it won't be long before you give up completely and a year passes you by. There will always be something on the horizon that will make you feel as if you need to put off starting: 'I'll start training on Monday because I'm wrecked after a week of work and I want to go out this weekend and enjoy myself' or 'I want to eat better, but I'm going out for dinner later, so I'll start tomorrow.' If you have this sort of attitude, then you're building on weak foundations.

There is no such thing as the perfect moment to begin your programme. So enough with the excuses and the external factors that you think are holding you back. Nothing is going to just fall into place for you. You have to decide what it is you want, then go out and make it happen on your own. Blah, blah, blah – just go work out!

"Blah, blah, blah – just go work out!"

Recognize your strengths

How many times have you heard someone say that they're not really good at anything? That statement is absolutely false, no matter who says it. We all have different skill sets and abilities, and once you realize that, you can begin to approach your goals from a much smarter angle. Make a list of what it is you think you're good at and back yourself up on it. 'I'm a good reader of people. I'm often approached by others for advice. I work well on a team. I'm actually pretty strong! I can think on my feet. I'm good at my job. I have great flexibility. I make an epic lasagne. I can't run for long, but I'm a really fast sprinter.'

Having confidence in your abilities is key, so acknowledge your strengths. Being aware of what you're good at isn't being cocky. If you only acknowledge your weaknesses and never remind yourself of your strengths, your outlook will become increasingly negative. This all relates back to a healthy fitness mindset. Give yourself a pat on the back every time you achieve a milestone. You can't be bad at eating right and training – anyone can do it, at varying levels.

Set goals

Imagine you set a goal and then told yourself that it's going to be impossible or really hard to achieve it. Do you think this would make things easier or more difficult? This goes back to visualizing exactly what it is you want to achieve. Outline your big goals, then decide what smaller goals you hope to achieve along the path to success. Start telling yourself 'I'm doing it' or 'I can do this, I've got this.' What's the point in thinking that the goal you've set for yourself is unobtainable? How can you reach your goal if you don't believe that you can do it?

By constantly reminding yourself that you have the ability to achieve your goals, you will subconsciously build up your confidence to the point where nothing will seem impossible. Tell yourself that you're already there. Act like you've conquered your dreams. This will feed your ambition because in your head you will know that you're not quite there yet, but in your heart you'll know that it's only just out of reach.

"Now is the time to train. Get in, get it done, get out."

Get into a routine

Routine will provide a structure to your life. Without routine, people end up feeling lost, sporadic and chaotic. I believe routine is one of the secrets to success, no matter what you're striving for. Even though I travel all the time, my days tend to follow the same pattern. I like to train at specific times, eat at specific times and work at specific times. For me, putting it in writing really helps. I keep a personal planner where I map out everything I'll be doing and hoping to achieve. I use it to help me to visualize what's coming up and begin to plan for how I'll approach certain situations. It also helps me to chart my goals. There's nothing more satisfying than putting a line through something I've accomplished.

By allocating a task to a specific time, you diminish the urge to procrastinate. Now is the time to train. Get in, get it done, get out. Now is the time to eat. Get your healthy, nutritious meal on, eat it and enjoy it. I try to apply the same mentality to everything I plan for: now is the time for this, so I'm going to focus all my energy on it, then move on to the next thing. Without a plan, I would feel as if I was spreading myself too thin and trying to juggle too much.

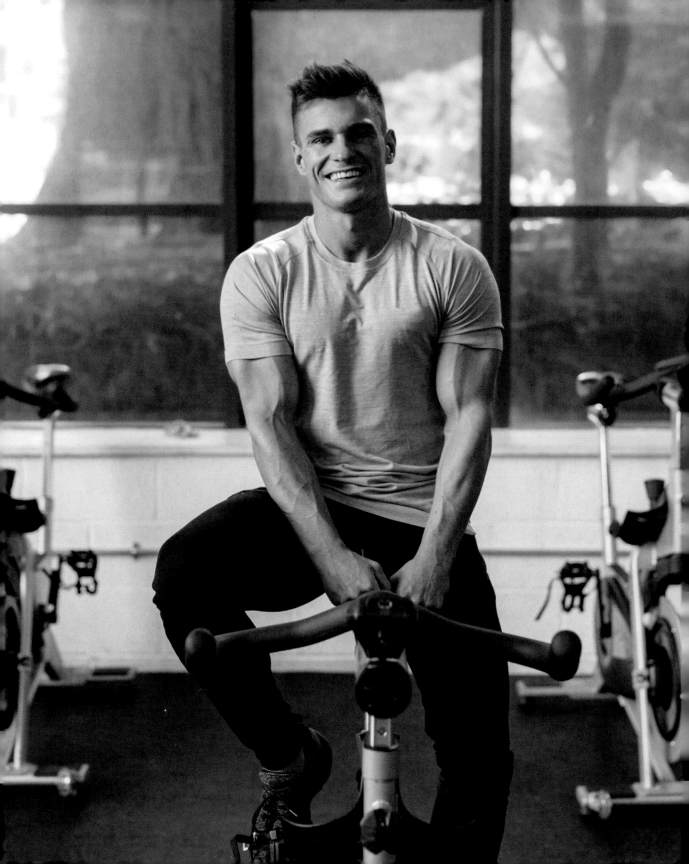

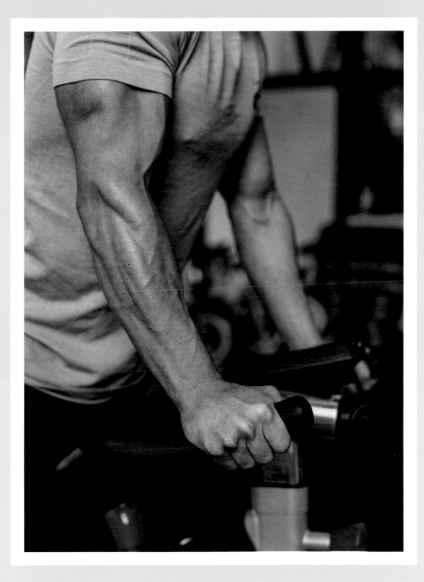

Stay calm

If something isn't going to plan, don't panic. We've all been there. Suddenly, you're faced with a struggle and you begin to imagine the worst-case scenario and the world becomes a much scarier place than it was five minutes ago. Your reaction in these moments is very important. Nothing is a problem — try to remove that word from your vocabulary. Try to think of problems as obstacles that need to be overcome rather than roadblocks that stop you from moving forward. Stay cool, take time to think, reassure yourself and move on.

Realize that failure is okay

> " You are going to fail. Failure is okay."

You are going to fail. Failure is okay. Repeat it. You are going to fail. Failure is okay. This is probably one of the most important things you need to tell yourself. Failure happens in many different ways and sometimes you might feel like all you're doing is failing. So if you don't meet your goals in a certain week or if you fall off the nutrition wagon and binge on pizza on a Wednesday, repeat this mantra. Try to change the word failure to 'progress'. Tell yourself that you are *learning* from your mistakes, not *failing*. Try to be a person you'd admire for trying rather than a victim who has decided that the universe has a vendetta against them and quits.

"

Dealing with
rejection is
a hugely
important
step towards
success."

Learn how to handle rejection

I had to include this one even though it doesn't directly relate to training and nutrition (well, the laughing at yourself bit does). It's such an important principle of mine that I want to convert you too. Dealing with rejection is a hugely important step towards success. We all get rejected in so many ways and at various points in our lives. It doesn't mean there is anything wrong with us — it just means that certain opportunities weren't right for us at that given moment.

If you allow your rejection to be a reflection of who you are, you will do nothing but create a negative outlook on your existence. Think of all the amazing actors you know who went for famous roles but didn't get them. Does that mean they're not good actors? Of course not. It just means they weren't right for the part. It's as simple as that. The word 'no' doesn't mean you aren't worthy, it just means that someone else can't see your potential. It's not you. Remind yourself of that. Don't let your abilities be defined by someone else. How can they possibly know your worth? Only you can know that. So when that moment of rejection comes, say, 'Thank you,' and come back even harder and stronger than before.

Be able to laugh at yourself

Laughing at yourself might not sound like much fun, but we Irish have the most wonderful ability to not take ourselves too seriously. The butt of a joke at home is often someone we love, and that person's participation in the joke only enhances the laughter. If you can't laugh at yourself, then what can you laugh at? By not taking yourself too seriously, you allow others to enjoy your company. If you do something stupid, try to laugh at it instead of becoming embarrassed by it. If you become paranoid over having made a fool of yourself, you'll never be happy. We all make complete fools of ourselves sometimes, but by laughing along with others you get to enjoy the moment rather than letting it haunt you. It's just another tool to use in the gym when you mess up an exercise or feel a little out of place.

> "You are you, so just focus on being the best version of you. Never worry about how that version measures up to somebody else."

Stop caring what other people think

People who say bad things about you or try to make you feel bad about yourself usually have a chip on their shoulder about something. Instead of responding to their toxicity, just leave them to it and let them drown in a pool of their own negativity. You don't need them or their pointless opinions.

Caring about what other people think of you can be a slippery slope to feeling bad about who you are. We live in an age where almost everything we do is (voluntarily) documented on social media. However, what you see on social media isn't the truth. For example, who posts pictures of themselves during their down times or when they're upset and dealing with something? Nobody. What you see on somebody's social media is their highlight reel, as chosen by them. You also might not see the years of work it took an individual to get to where they are, so don't compare your Chapter 1 to someone else's Chapter 10.

Basically, it's a nice boost to get praise for something and it's never nice to be criticized, but the only opinion I truly care about is my own because I'm the only person who has to live with my own thoughts and feelings. If you keep comparing yourself to other people, you'll quickly suffocate under your own feelings of inadequacy. You are you, so just focus on being the best version of you. Never worry about how that version measures up to somebody else.

Stop complaining

You've got two choices when something doesn't go your way: give in and wonder why it's always you who's shit out of luck or brush it off as another lesson learned. Nobody wants to be around negative people. Negativity sucks the life out of everything and frankly is a boring downer. If you complain instead of working out how a situation can be improved, all you're doing is wasting time and creating a toxic environment.

There is a difference between getting something off your chest and moaning incessantly until others are sick of listening to you. Yes, you might be experiencing a tough time, but do you honestly believe that giving out about it is going to make it better? I'm not saying that frustration is a bad thing, but it's how you deal with frustration that will define the outcome of your predicament. Use the energy created by your anger and channel it into something positive. Go for a fast walk with your favourite music turned up loud or hit the gym and smash out some reps — that way, you're making your frustration work in your favour.

Recognize the things that don't matter

This follows on from the complaining trap above. Getting hung up on irrelevant details or worrying about past events that you can do nothing about will get you nowhere. There are so many little things in life that we give weight to that really mean nothing in the grand scheme of things. I once had a teacher at school who advised us to write down everything we were worried about and to not look at our list for a year. He said that if we did it, we'd laugh at what we'd written down a year later. I don't remember what I wrote down, but he was right.

We so often allow minor details to become big worries that loom over us like dark, heavy clouds. Freeing yourself of such worries gives you the power to focus on what's most important in your life. Ask yourself, 'Do I really care about this? Is this important to my long-term goals? Am I going to let this influence my life?'

> "Use the energy created by your anger and channel it into something positive."

THE ROB LIPSETT GAME PLAN

Stay positive

Positivity breeds positivity. Negativity breeds negativity. If you approach a scenario with a positive mindset, you'll take something positive from it, no matter what the outcome is. You failed? No — you learned, you grew. This sort of attitude will help you to identify exactly what it is you need to do in order to succeed. Having a negative approach to something just sets you up for a negative experience. It makes you want to give up, and then when you do fail it validates what you already expected. A big waste of time all round.

Have fun

I know, I know, it sounds simplistic to tell you to just have fun when things may be going badly for you, but believe me, having fun is so important! Striking a balance between fun and work allows us to grow and progress. Of course, we think we would all love it if life was one big party, but I don't think we would. Enjoying the fruits of your labour is half the satisfaction of achieving your goals. You earned this, you deserve this, you made this possible.

It's a given that you have to put your head down and work hard if you're going to succeed. However, you also need to step back and strike a balance between work and play. Without balance, our lives would be nothing but excess. So yes, it's admirable that you work your ass off day in and day out, but take some time to enjoy yourself with people you like. The same thing applies to the gym — there's no point being in great shape, working out 24/7, if your life is one-dimensional and you never see any friends or have any fun.

When you are having fun, go all in. Try not to worry about the things going on in your life that might be bothering you. Now is the time to enjoy yourself — later is for hard work and perseverance. The same goes for when you're hard at work. Give it your all, because later on is going to taste so sweet when you can relax. This tenet applies to the work you do to earn a crust and the work you do in the gym to reach your body goals. I stress the importance of enjoying your training later in the book (see page 114). Don't do a routine three times a week that does your head in and feels like a constant chore — find exercises you enjoy doing.

> "There's no point being in great shape, working out 24/7, if your life is one-dimensional and you never see any friends or have any fun."

Bust out of your comfort zone and be open-minded

There's a lot of research out there right now that advocates the positive mental effects of challenging yourself, leaving your comfort zone and doing something that actually creates a small frisson of fear. This doesn't mean that you should watch horror films to the point that you're sleeping with the light on, or hurl yourself out of a plane or go heli-skiing in the Alps. The thing is, comfort can quickly become laziness. If you're not going into situations that make you nervous, excited or scared, then you're doing nothing but coasting by. Nerves are good; being scared is good. It means you care. This can apply to physical challenges (which is where we're headed in this book), business challenges or stuff in your personal life, like asking that person out for a coffee.

You might find yourself thinking, 'Oh God, what have I let myself in for?' or 'I hope this works out.' These thoughts are good for you. If you didn't think this way sometimes, then how boring would your life be? I would never want to live like that. I've been scared so many times in my life by making big decisions because what I was doing felt like a big step. When I posted my first YouTube video, I had a panic attack after I'd pressed the publish button! Same when I started my first business. But I tried to harness those nerves and use them, and so far it's worked pretty well. However, you've got to keep a bit of that fear — if I didn't feel nervous or scared before big moments, I'd start to worry. It would mean that I didn't care enough.

Stay open to new experiences throughout your life, whether you're 25 or 75. For example, if you're a picky eater, you don't have to go out and try brains or ox tongue, but don't limit yourself. Start small. Nobody wants to be the chicken-nuggets-and-chips kid forever. By refusing to try new things, you're limiting your ability to learn. So many amazing opportunities in life can pass you by if you say no to everything. You'll surprise yourself if you have an open outlook and are willing to let new experiences present themselves to you. One of my favourite quotes about life comes from Oscar Wilde, who said, 'Nothing that is worth knowing can be taught.' It's so true. Until you go out and experience something for yourself, you can't fully understand it.

"When I posted my first YouTube video, I had a panic attack after I'd pressed the publish button!"

Put in 100 per cent

This is one of the most important factors in your mindset reboot to prepare yourself for what's ahead in this book. If you really want what you've set out to achieve, then you must realize that none of it is going to come easy. There will be times when your patience will be seriously tested, as will your ability to dig deep and keep going. Sometimes you'll find yourself wondering if it's really worth it — the discipline, the time commitment, the meal planning, the lack (or reduction) of certain well-loved but unhealthy treats, the sweat, the aches . . . but that's when you need to keep going. The pursuit of your goals will seriously test your resolve, but when you overcome hurdles and feel the satisfaction of success you'll know that your efforts were worth it, every single time.

"If you really want what you've set out to achieve, then you must realize that none of it is going to come easy."

TAKE-HOME POINTS

> Start small and build up your fitness gradually, otherwise you'll burn out and get nowhere.

> There's no perfect time to start your fitness and nutrition journey, so banish those excuses and stop putting things off until all the stars are in alignment.

> Identify your strengths and recognize that we all have them.

> Set specific goals and visualize yourself having reached them already.

> Make a routine and stick to it. Have your plan set for the week and don't diverge from it.

> Think of problems as obstacles instead of roadblocks and you will climb over them.

> Accept that you're going to fail occasionally and that it's okay.

> Learn to handle rejection and laugh at yourself with grace and verve.

> Don't worry about what people think or compare yourself to others. Just focus on being the best version of you.

> Don't waste time complaining. It's annoying, and you can channel that energy into something positive.

> Look at the bigger picture — don't sweat the small stuff.

> Have fun when you're working, working out and playing.

> Regularly try new things that challenge you and are outside your comfort zone.

> Understand that you will have to put in huge amounts of effort at times to get what you want to achieve.

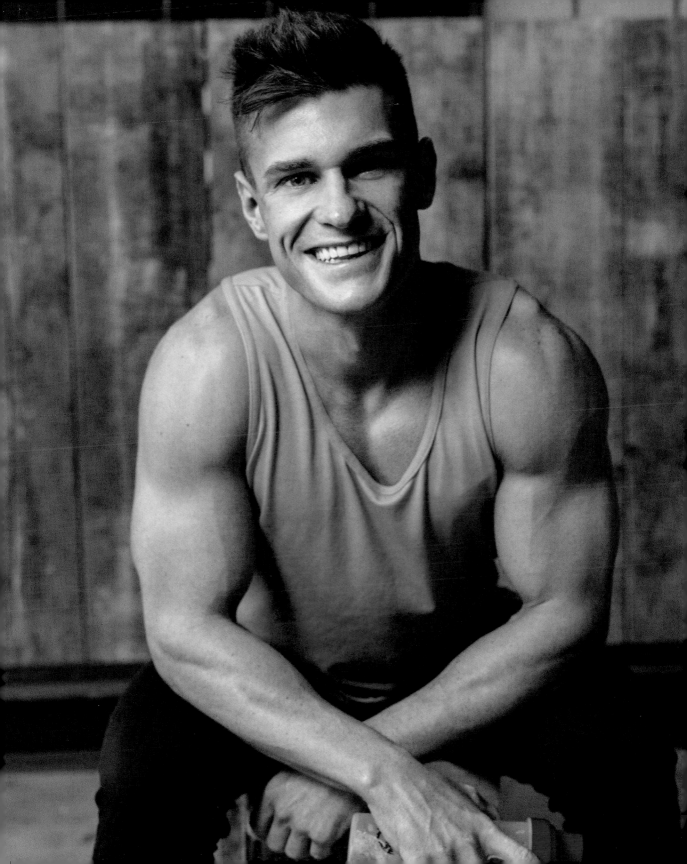

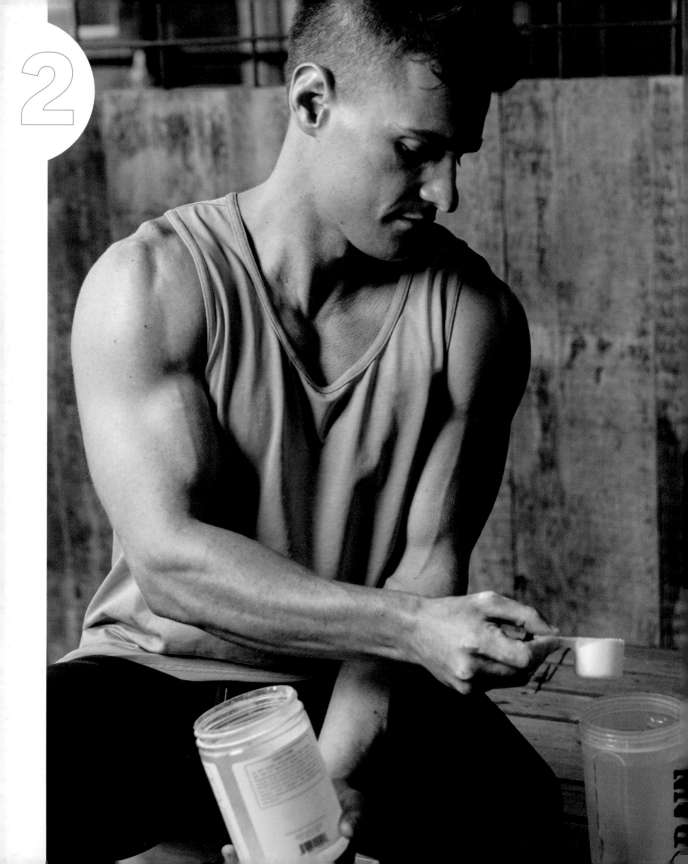

2

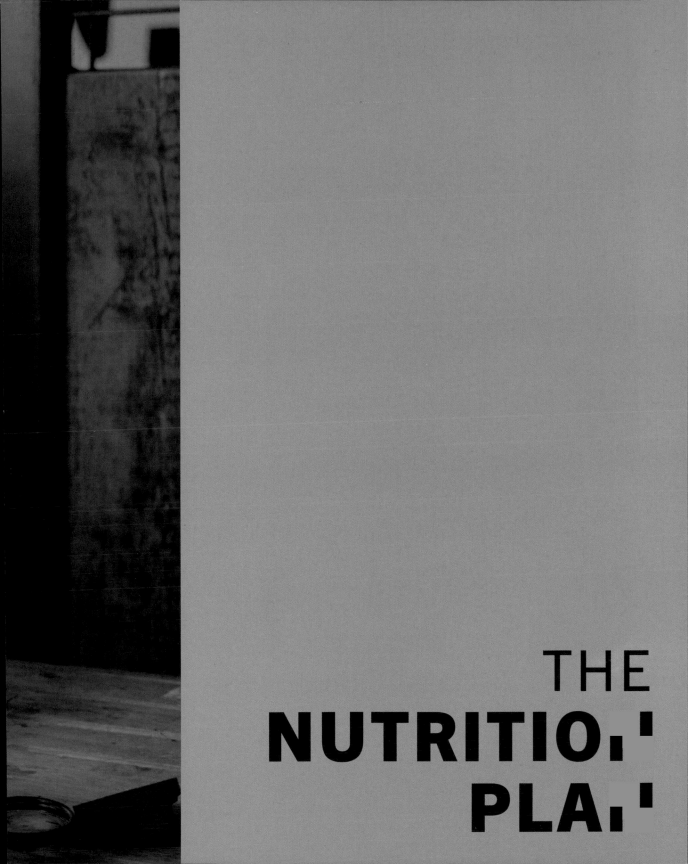

THE
NUTRITIO.'
PLA.'

THE NUTRITION PLAN

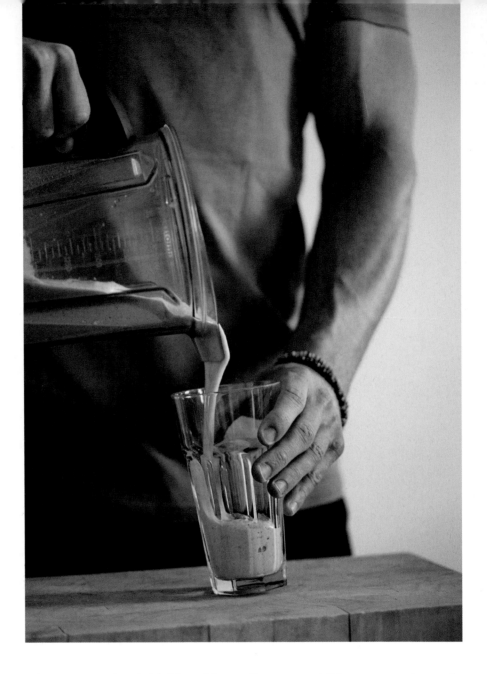

What you eat (and drink) and how often you eat it is a cornerstone of getting into great shape — that and sustained training, which we'll get into in the next chapter. All this means a lot to me, so sharing it with you has a much deeper meaning than just teaching you how to track your meals and prep nutritious food in advance so that you don't get caught out and have to compromise and eat stuff that's not going to do you any favours. This is the stuff that changed my life.

Set up your diet

Let me start by saying that what I'm going to present you with are *guidelines*, not personalized diet plans. But they will still make for a great starting point and you can adjust things as time goes on. When it comes to diet, nothing beats trial and error and learning how to listen to your body.

> **THE KEY TO MANIPULATING YOUR BODY COMPOSITION IS YOUR CALORIE/MACRONUTRIENT INTAKE.**

"It doesn't matter if you don't count calories: calories still count."

Remember those words. We've all heard of calories, but *macronutrient* is a fancy word for the type of food we eat: protein, fats and carbohydrates. You can go low carb, gluten free, paleo, vegan, sugar free, fat free or whatever fad appeals, but if you are not in a caloric *deficit* (burning more than you take in), you are not going to lose fat. Full stop. It doesn't matter if you don't count calories: calories still count. People don't like to hear that harsh reality and there are many fitness gurus out there who will try to tell you that calories don't matter, but that is not what I'm about. I'm about keeping it real, as I've said at the end of every single YouTube video I've ever made. And people appreciate that honesty.

So what approach do you take if you want to lose fat? You need to find a plan that gets you results and allows you to sustain that caloric deficit. Then you need to stick to that plan. A calorie is a unit of energy. Fat is simply stored energy. To lose the fat, you need to be taking in less energy than you're expending. Let me slow down for a second with the science and spell it all out.

MACRONUTRIENTS = protein, carbohydrates and fats.

These are what make up your calories.

- **1G OF PROTEIN** = 4 calories
- **1G OF CARBOHYDRATE** = 4 calories
- **1G OF FAT** = 9 calories

These figures don't change. Whether you're getting protein from a steak or a shake, 1g of protein will always equal 4 calories. Picture a building with several storeys: the calories are the foundations and the macronutrients are the floors. They are inextricably linked! By tracking macronutrients, you are also tracking calories by default. For example, if you increase or decrease your carbs, you're also increasing or decreasing your calorie intake. It all goes back to the numbers above.

When people cut a certain macronutrient, such as carbohydrates, from their diet and lose weight, they say it must have been the carbs that were making them fat, but this isn't the case. It was the *calories* from the carbs that were making them fat! The same goes for something like gluten or wheat. People remove gluten, wheat or another significant food that they usually eat from their diet and end up excluding a lot of *calorie-dense food* (pasta, bread, cereal, etc.). It's the same scenario – reducing the calories that those foods contain makes people lose the weight, not specifically reducing the bread or the pasta. All diets are essentially the same but are dressed up differently. They all serve to reduce your calorie intake, whether or not you're aware of it.

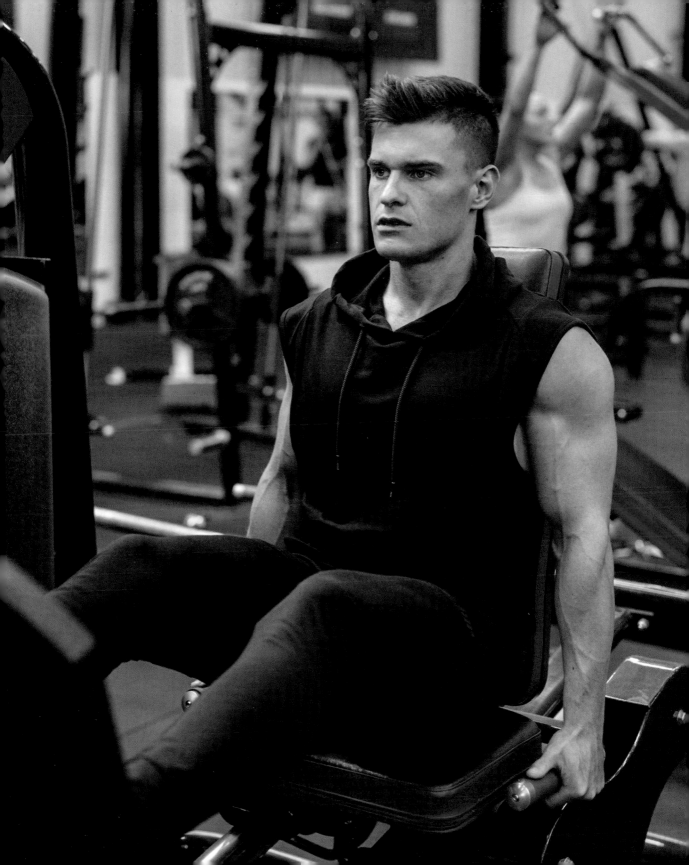

Total daily energy expenditure (TDEE)

Your total daily energy expenditure (TDEE) is simply how many calories (energy) your body uses/needs every day. Working this out is an important step in planning a diet that is tailored to the unique way in which your body works.

Now, a bit of background before you run for the hills with all this science – believe me, it will all make sense eventually! Our bodies use calories for a lot of things, including:

- Staying alive: your basal metabolic rate (BMR)
- Daily tasks like sitting down and standing up: non-exercise-activated thermogenesis (NEAT)
- Digesting the food you eat: thermic effect of food (TEF)

Figuring out your TDEE is the only thing you need to think about – it's your total daily energy expenditure, with *total* being the key word here. Looking up 'calorie/ TDEE calculator' on the internet and plugging in a few simple stats will give you an accurate enough reading. I recommend you try a few different calculators and take an average. You will also need to plug in lifestyle factors. For example, if you have a sedentary desk job you'll have a very different TDEE compared to someone who works on a building site. Another option is to multiply your weight in pounds by 15–16 for a female or by 17–18 for a male.

I should stress that the methods above are just the starting point. As I said earlier, trial and error is king in this business. Metabolisms can vary a bit and we all know someone who can eat whatever they want and stay slim (annoying, I know!).

After you've figured out how many calories you need daily (maintenance), track your intake for a week or two. Weigh yourself *every morning* before eating or drinking and after going to the bathroom for the most accurate reading. It's better to get a weekly average, as you can have quick jumps or decreases in body weight from day to day. If your weight stays the same or changes very little, then you've successfully worked out your maintenance calories/TDEE. If it goes up or down, you'll need to tweak your intake until you find your perfect maintenance calories.

> "Trial and error is king in this business."

Meeting your goals

Now that you've done the figures and you're satisfied that you know how many calories you should be taking in per day, it's time to examine your goal in this process. Is it to:

- Lose body fat and get lean?
- Increase your weight and focus on building muscle?
- Maintain the physique you already have? (This is the end goal for most people.)

> "You can't pay someone else to do the work for you."

I get asked all the time how I stay in shape and stay lean all year round, and I'm here to tell you that there is no shortcut. It's about discipline, putting in the work and knowing how your body works, through and through. You can't pay someone else to do the work for you.

Since the starting point for many of you reading this book is probably to drop body fat and get lean, let's start there. A general guideline is to go around 500 calories below the TDEE that you've calculated, trialled for a while and tweaked to your satisfaction. One pound of fat comes to about 3,500 calories, so if you eat 500 calories less than your TDEE per day, you're looking at one pound of fat loss per week. This is the ideal rate of weight loss to aim for, as it allows you to keep both your muscle and your strength — and, importantly, your sanity too. Losing weight too quickly isn't the way to go, as your muscle will be lost too. If this happens, you can introduce a 'cheat day' once a week where you eat more calories to get back on the right track.

On the other hand, if you cut down too little, your diet could last for months and months with little result and frustration will set in. If you get into a good routine and develop good habits, then sticking to your plan will become effortless. I've seen this happen to clients all the time. After the initial teething period at the beginning of a plan, things get easier.

If you want to *add* muscle and bulk, you do the opposite and consume 200–300 calories above your TDEE.

TAKE-HOME POINTS

> STEP 1:

Estimate your maintenance calories by using online calculators or by multiplying your body weight in pounds by 15–16 for females and 17–18 for males. Use the higher number if you're active and train regularly.

> STEP 2:

Track your weight for a week or two and see how your body responds to find your true maintenance calorie figure.

- If fat loss is your goal, consume 300–500 calories below your maintenance level.

- If lean muscle/weight gain is the goal, consume 200–300 calories above your maintenance level.

- Decide on one approach – fat loss or gaining muscle/weight – and stick to it. When people try to do both, they often just end up going nowhere or getting slow results.

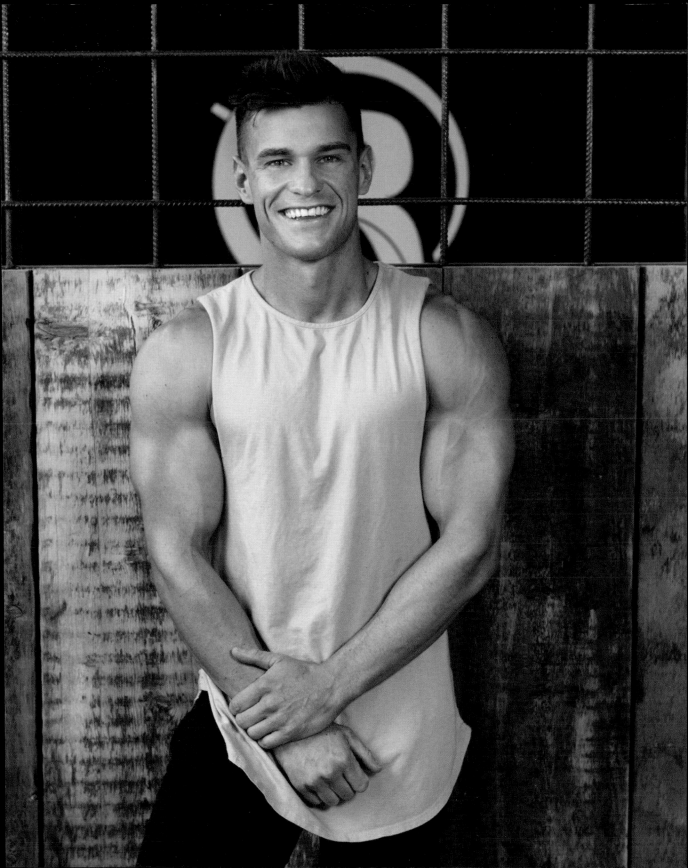

How to calculate macronutrients

One of my main aims in this book is to keep things as simple as possible and not bore you with science, but I do need to go into more detail on calories and macronutrients. They are so important in health and physique that I just can't leave them out, so bear with me.

As I mentioned earlier, macronutrients (macros for short) are what make up our calories. They are the three types of food: protein, fat and carbohydrate (see page 40 for how they translate to calories). Calorie intake determines whether weight is gained or lost, but it's the macronutrients that influence whether that change in weight is from fat or muscle mass. As an example, imagine that two people were put on diets where they could each consume 2,500 calories a day, but one of them had to eat only fats to make up the calories. You don't need to be a rocket scientist to guess that they will look and perform very differently from the person whose caloric intake consists of a good mix of carbs, protein and fats.

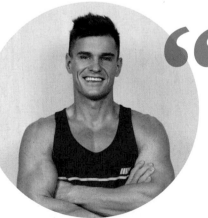

"If you get into a good routine and develop good habits, then sticking to your plan will become effortless."

Let's go into a bit more detail about these three nutrients . . .

1. PROTEIN

Protein is vital for life. The body breaks protein down into its building blocks, essential amino acids. Protein helps us gain muscle and avoid muscle breakdown, aids recovery and healing, helps our immune system, stops us from feeling hungry and slows down our digestion rate. Protein is often thought of as the most important macronutrient when it comes to our body composition. Protein-rich foods include meat, eggs and fish.

2. FATS

The idea of fats being one of the essential nutrients may be surprising. Fats have been given a bad name by the serial abuse of the 'wrong' kinds of fats (think deep-fried Mars bars or battered sausages), which is causing all kinds of health problems worldwide. Yet the truth is that the 'right' kinds of fats consumed in the right way for health provide our bodies with essential fatty acids. These keep our hormones functioning correctly, providing us with important vitamins and minerals and aid general health. Examples of fat-rich foods include full-fat dairy products, certain meats, avocados and nuts (those last two will be easily recognized as health guru staples!).

3. CARBOHYDRATES

Carbohydrates are not classed as an *essential* nutrient, but I think you can argue this case. They are our bodies' preferred energy source, as they are really easy to break down and convert into fuel in the form of glucose (more about that later). They are needed for the brain, kidney, muscles and heart to function properly and they also add to your fibre intake, which not only keeps your gut healthy but can also keep you feeling fuller for longer. There is also research to show that carbohydrates help fuel your workouts, which in turn allows you to perform better and avoid muscle loss when getting lean. Carbohydrate-rich foods include potatoes, pasta, bread and oats, but they are also found in lesser amounts in vegetables, beans and pulses.

Daily macronutrient guidelines

Here are my guidelines when it comes to setting the right daily targets with your macronutrients:

- **PROTEIN: 0.8–1.2g per pound of body weight**
- **FATS: 0.3–0.5g per pound of body weight or 20 per cent of your total calorie intake**
- **CARBOHYDRATES: These can make up the remainder of your calorie intake**

If you find yourself feeling too hungry at any point in your plan, you could increase the amount of protein, as this will help with the hunger pangs and also preserve lean tissue when in a deficit. You can play around with the ratios of carbs and fats too (lower carb/higher fat or higher fat/lower carb). Get to know your body and experiment to see what works best for you.

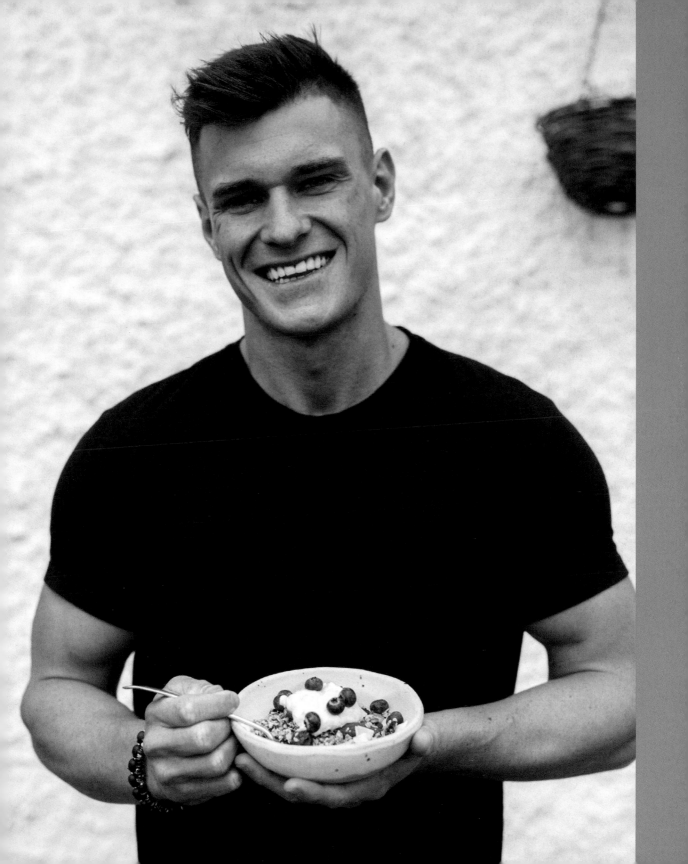

Examples of foods in the macronutrient groups

PROTEIN	CARBOHYDRATES	FATS	VEGETABLES & FRUITS
Chicken	Basmati rice	Almonds	Asparagus
Egg whites	Beans	Avocado	Broccoli
Ham	Bran cereal	Cashews	Brussels sprouts
High-protein	Brown rice	Coconut oil	Cabbage
milk	Lentils	Natural peanut	Carrots
Lean beef	Oatmeal	butter	Cauliflower
Low-fat Greek	Potatoes	Olive oil	Celery
yoghurt	Quinoa	Organic butter	Courgettes
Mackerel	Sweet potato	Organic milk	Cucumbers
Prawns	Wholewheat	Walnuts	Garlic
Salmon	bread	Whole eggs	Green beans
Tuna	Wholewheat		Kale
Turkey	pasta		Lettuce
			Mushrooms
			Onions
			Pak choi
			Peppers
			Spinach
			Tomatoes
			Apples
			Bananas
			Blueberries
			Grapefruit
			Kiwi
			Oranges
			Pears
			Raspberries
			Strawberries

Black pepper
Cayenne
pepper
Chilli powder
Cinnamon
Garlic
Hot sauce
Light balsamic
vinegar
Light soy sauce
or tamari
Malt vinegar
Sea salt
Turmeric

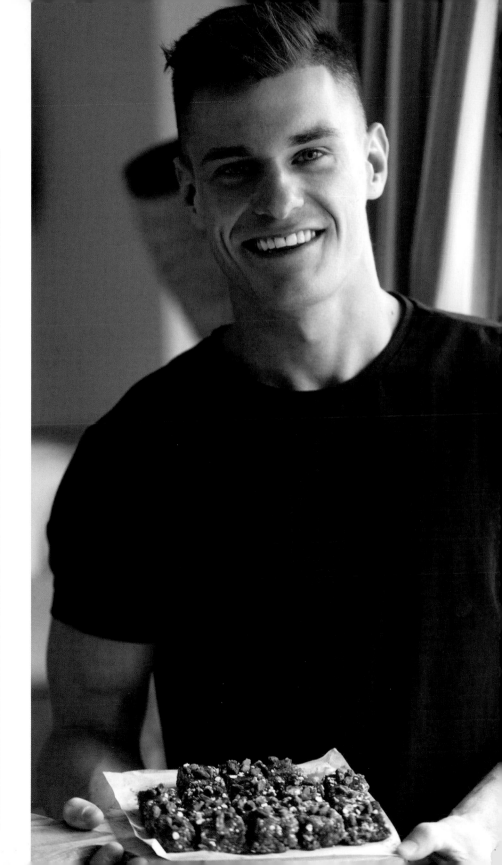

Low fat or low carb?

In the 1980s we thought that fat was the root of all evil, but now people are saying that insulin is what is making us fat or that we should eat paleo, like our prehistoric friends (um, newsflash: most people in the Paleolithic era died from starvation). We now have research-based evidence proving that there is no 'bad' macronutrient or food group — total energy balance will dictate whether or not you gain fat. But everyone is different in their response to diets. For example, those carrying more body fat tend to do better with a higher fat intake than leaner individuals; leaner people do better with a lower fat intake, while athletic people tend to do better on a higher-carb diet. Whatever approach you choose, make sure it's the easiest one to stick to. If you can't hack it day to day, then it's pointless.

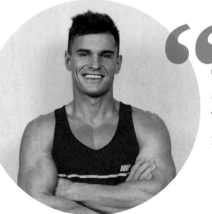

"There is no 'bad' macronutrient or food group — total energy balance will dictate whether or not you gain fat."

TAKE-HOME POINTS

> Set your protein intake first, then set your carb and fat intakes: low carb, low fat or a mixture of both. Find out what suits you and what you can stick to.

> Set your protein intake at 0.8–1.2g per pound of body weight. The higher end of the range is suggested for those who are deep-cutting calories, more advanced trainees or those who struggle with appetite.

> Set your fat intake at 0.3–0.5g per pound of body weight or limit it to 20 per cent of your total calorie intake.

> If you're overweight, use your lean body weight (your weight minus the fat) for these calculations.

> Allocate the remainder of your calories to carbs or swap between fats and carbs if you prefer.

> The main thing is net calories and net protein intake, so it's important to choose a macronutrient split that you can adhere to.

You have to start with the tracking or you'll never hack the intuitive eating."

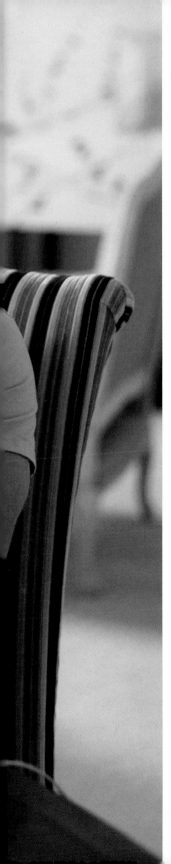

How to track your macronutrient/ calorie intake

So how do you track your macronutrient/calorie intake? Don't worry, it doesn't have to be complicated: all you need is a good digital kitchen scales and a smartphone. Download a macro/calorie/food diary app on your phone (I recommend MyFitnessPal), then log *everything* you eat and drink for the next few weeks. Drinks other than water can contain huge amounts of calories, so be mindful of this. Don't be put off by this commitment – spending a few *minutes* each day to log your meals will save you *weeks* of frustration and wondering why the results you had hoped for aren't happening!

Make sure you log the correct brand or type of food into your diary. For example, different cuts of beef will contain different amounts of fat. By the same token, one brand of Greek yoghurt could have added sugar/carbs or less protein than another brand and one type of peanut butter could have added oils compared to another. This really applies to everything, so be specific – there's no point doing this if you're not. So if it's Tesco yoghurt, enter 100g Tesco Greek yoghurt. If it's Aldi peanut butter, enter 30g Aldi smooth/crunchy peanut butter.

What about veggies and very low-calorie foods? Do they need to be logged too? Only if you are in serious competition training, where every calorie counts. For most of us, there's no need to do this. You'll get results just from making better food choices and developing better eating habits.

It might sound obvious, but another important thing to bear in mind is that you need to be brutally honest in your diary. There are so many studies that show that people estimate they're eating hundreds of calories less than what they're actually eating. Not accounting for every single thing you're eating means you're wasting your time.

I know that tracking your food can be boring, but I'm not asking you to do it for the rest of your life! After you've done it for a few weeks, you'll have a much better understanding of portions and what a serving of food looks like. When you've become more attuned to your appetite, you'll be able to try out intuitive eating, which is a stress-free way to eat according to how you feel. But you can't learn to run before walking, so you have to start with the tracking or you'll never hack the intuitive eating.

TAKE-HOME POINTS

> **DOWNLOAD** MyFitnessPal or the macro-tracking app of your choice and buy a set of digital kitchen scales.

> **READ** food labels.

> **BE PRECISE** with your tracking, especially for the first few weeks, to get a good idea of exactly what you're taking in.

> The lower the body-fat percentage you want to get to, the more precisely you'll need to monitor your food intake.

> Further down the line you can taper off from tracking while still maintaining the good habits and portion control that you learned from doing it.

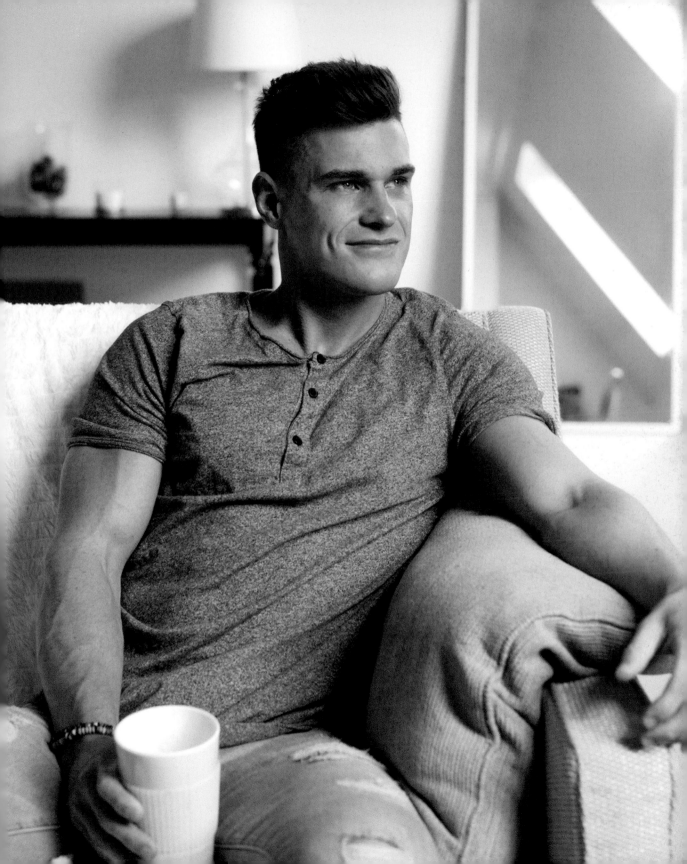

How to monitor your progress

When it comes to getting the best out of your tracking and ensuring it's as accurate as it can be, the magic word is consistency. Let's have a look at a few ways to monitor your progress.

1. SCALE WEIGHT

Weigh yourself every morning when you wake up, before eating or drinking anything and after you go to the bathroom. Make sure you always wear the same type of thing — or nothing — each time or your numbers won't be accurate. I advise taking a weekly average and not focusing on a daily number. Scale numbers can mess with your head and there are so many factors that can affect them — here are just a few (some may surprise you!):

- Carb intake
- Water intake
- Salt/sodium intake
- Water retention (when too much fluid has built up in the body)
- Stress (if scale weight stresses you out, weigh yourself less often)
- A bad sleep
- The time of your last meal
- Food still being digested, even if you ate it hours ago (some foods, such as red meat, take a really long time to digest)
- Bowel movements (could mean less or more on the scale number)

2. PROGRESS PICTURES

Some people won't like this idea (and I know I'm no shrinking violet when it comes to the selfies!), but progress pictures are an important way to monitor your progress. Take your picture at the same time (perhaps after your weigh-in) in the same spot with the same lighting each time. You don't need to do this every day — once a week or fortnightly is ideal, as that way you'll be more likely to notice progress. If you fancy posting your progress pics on social media, go for it! Some people find it fun and that it keeps them accountable.

3. GYM PROGRESS

Keep an eye on your progress in the gym if you train there regularly. If you're losing pounds and are able to lift heavier weights, that's awesome. But if you don't seem to have enough strength to have a good workout, you might need to increase your calories.

4. MEASUREMENTS

Measuring key areas of the body can be a great way to monitor your progress, especially for beginners who may be building muscle and losing fat at the same time. In these cases, you may be stepping on the scales daily and seeing no change, which is disheartening, but it's likely that you're still losing fat. Physically taking fat measurements can solve this frustration. As it's much more fiddly than just stepping on the scales, I wouldn't recommend doing this more than once a month.

Key areas to measure with your measuring tape are:

- Arms
- Chest
- Hips
- Midsection
- Thighs
- Waist

Meal planning

I'll start this off by saying that I'm not a huge fan of rigid meal plans, as they take away the autonomy of doing your own food tracking. There's also the problem of the mindset that comes with being on a rigid plan. If someone eats something that's not on their meal plan, they might think, 'Screw it, I messed up. Time to order a wagon wheel stuffed-crust pizza with a side of wedges and a gallon of Sprite!' Added to this is the difficulty of sticking to a meal plan when you're travelling, eating out, going to a party, etc.

That said, meal plans can add structure to your routine and can help you to develop good eating habits since you don't have to put as much thought into what to make for your next meal. Meal plans dished out by the hardcore bodybuilder in your local gym won't take into account what you like or don't like, so my solution is to build your own meal plan that includes the foods you like.

- **TRACK your macros with *full accuracy* for five days.**

- **WRITE down everything you ate *in the order that you ate it*.**

- **BOOM! You now have five meal plans catered to your tastes. It's as simple as that.**

Flexible dieting

A myth I'd like to debunk right here is that some foods are 'bad'. There is no such thing as 'good' and 'bad' *foods* — there are only good and bad *diets*. It's possible to have a good diet that contains 'bad' food and vice versa. Are you having a single slice of pizza while walking through town with a friend or are you ordering a large pizza all for yourself twice a week? Without knowing the context, we can't just say that pizza is 'bad'.

Unfortunately, there will always be a health or fitness professional who will claim that a certain food is 'bad'. There are so many worthy brigades out there who have a lot to say about food — vegans, low-carbers, paleo fanatics, food pyramid promoters, the government, hippies, organic-only evangelists, you name it. I've even heard some nutters say we shouldn't have fats and carbs together on the same plate! Everyone is disagreeing with each other. Whatever the food or the food group, someone, somewhere, is telling us it's bad for our health. So I guess we should just eat air and water? Wait, I'm not sure what the current stance is on water . . .

This all-or-nothing approach is what gets people yo-yo dieting and bingeing. What's the solution? Enter flexible dieting, which is a more balanced approach. Here's an example to put it in context. Say you're cutting down, with a 2,000-calorie-a-day diet. You go to the cinema and can't resist treating yourself to a Snickers bar, which contains about 250 calories. What do you think would be the best way to handle having this treat?

1 BE THE DIE-HARD CLEAN EATER.
Eat the candy bar but feel guilty and ashamed, then write the rest of the day off and buy a tub of ice cream on the way home too.

2 BE THE FLEXIBLE DIETER.
Eat the candy bar and enjoy it without feeling guilty because you realize that it didn't even impact your overall calorie intake for the day.

Which person do you think will be more successful in developing healthy eating habits and meeting their dietary goals in the long run?

'Bad' foods — the foods that 'clean eaters' look down on — are only bad for you when they make up a large part of your diet and cause you to miss out on certain necessary nutrients. If 80–90 per cent of what you eat is nutrient-rich wholefood to get enough vitamins, minerals and fibre into you, then knock yourself out with some of your favourite treat foods. If you can't sustain your diet and enjoy a treat now and then, it simply won't last.

Is a carb always a carb?

I often get asked this type of question: 'Okay, so you've got your macros and calories worked out for fat loss and muscle gain, but surely carbs from a doughnut aren't the same as carbs from brown rice or a sweet potato?' The answer is actually yes *and* no.

Carbohydrates are usually classed into two types: **simple** and **complex**.

- **SIMPLE CARBS** have one or two sugars and are easily absorbed and broken down. They are a quick fix, giving you an energy boost soon after eating. Examples include fruit, fizzy drinks, cakes and biscuits.

- **COMPLEX CARBS** contain three or more sugars and take longer for the body to absorb, meaning you get a slower release of energy. Examples include oatmeal, potatoes and vegetables.

People tend to think that sugary carbs will make them fat, but studies have been done where all macronutrients are equated, yet one group eats a diet high in sugary carb sources and another eats a diet high in complex/starchy carb sources. Fat loss and markers on health are identical as long as the total carb intake is the same.

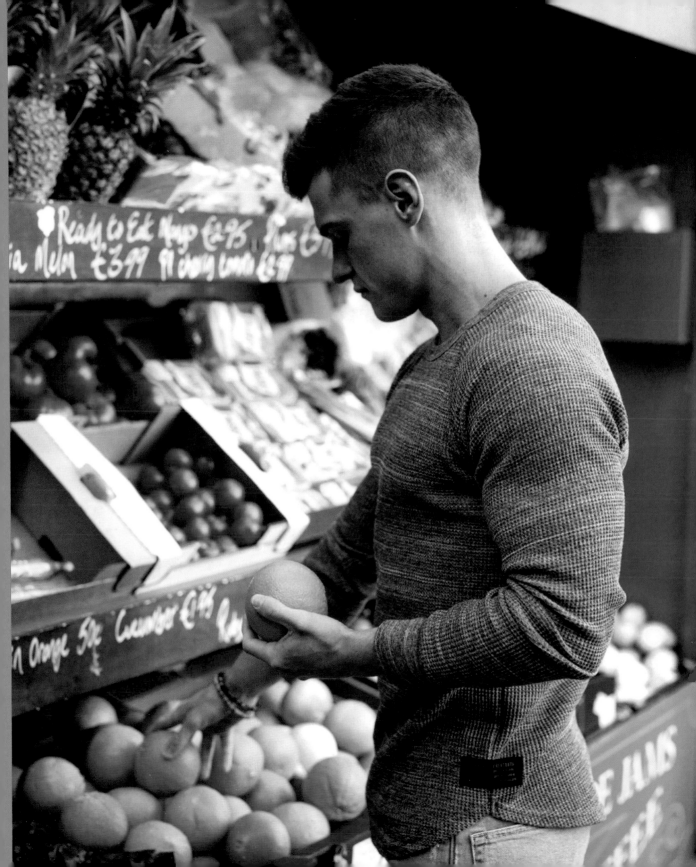

Hitting a fat-loss wall

You may be doing great on your plan, then suddenly notice that you don't seem to be losing fat any more. The mantra to reassure yourself with here is: *Fat loss is not linear.* Ironically, it's when you're doing really well, getting leaner and well into your diet, that things will start to slow down. Don't worry if you stall for a week but then pick up again. If that week turns into two weeks, though, it may be time to take some action. Here's my failsafe plan to get things going again.

1. TRACK MORE ACCURATELY

Number one on the list has to be to look at your food intake again (see page 55). As you get much leaner, your body can go into 'survival mode', because it thinks you are literally starving to death. In that kind of a situation, you'll reach out for food such as cheese and bread samples in the supermarket and your brain won't even register it. It may seem like such a small thing, but over a week this kind of stuff can really add up. Ask yourself if you're hitting your calorie/macro goals and be brutally honest.

2. MOVE MORE

This has nothing to do with the gym — it's about what you do *outside* the gym. Confused? There's this thing called NEAT (non-exercise-activated thermogenesis), which refers to the calories you burn when you're not exercising and are just going about your daily life. These are the calories you burn walking to the shop, climbing the stairs, hoovering the living room, that sort of thing. NEAT just happens, so once you become aware of it you can develop some good habits to promote it, such as taking the stairs instead of the lift or parking further away from your destination than you need to. The bonus? You'll end up burning a lot more calories throughout the week without even noticing. I often advise my clients who work in an office to stand up, stretch and walk to the cooler for a drink every 20–30 minutes. Imagine you burned an extra calorie every minute just by making that one simple change:

> Even if you don't count the calories, the calories still count."

8 hours x 60 calories

= 480 calories per day

= 2,400 per week!

3. STOP EATING OUT

Now I'm no party pooper and I think it's great to get out and sit round a table with your friends and family, but a restaurant chef's job is to make the food taste as good as possible, regardless of your fat-loss goals. A restaurant meal will almost certainly have a lot of added oils and sugars you're not aware of — think about the amount of butter and salt those TV chefs lash into everything! So if your progress has stalled, take a break from eating out and start prepping more of your own meals. I'll give you some tips on how to handle a night out later in the book (see page 104), but meanwhile, remember, even if you don't count the calories, the calories still count.

4. TAKE A DIET BREAK OR A REFEED

It may seem counter-intuitive, but taking a break from a diet can help to restart stalled weight loss. Dieting for a prolonged amount of time can be stressful and stress raises our cortisol levels (cortisol is often called the stress hormone), which causes us to hold on to a lot of water weight. In this situation, taking a diet break for a week or so (while returning to your maintenance calories; see page 42) or having a refeed (a day where you double your carb intake and 'carb up') can take some of this stress off. Suddenly you might drop the water weight and break through the plateau in what's called the 'whoosh' effect. Going back to maintenance calories for a while will also reset any negative things that may have occurred while dieting, such as mental fatigue with the whole thing. Think about it as taking one step back but two steps forward.

"Think about it as taking one step back but two steps forward."

5. MONITOR YOUR WEEKEND HABITS

Keep in mind that it's not just about your net daily energy balance, it's also the weekly balance — and that includes weekends. I often see people who eat 500 calories less per day during the week but then binge-eat at the weekend. When you add that into a daily average, it turns out they're not eating 500 calories less per day at all. This is why it's so important to pick a diet you can stick to and don't mind following (see page 52).

6. EMERGENCY MEASURES

If all of the above fails and your plateau still refuses to budge, then I recommend these emergency measures:

- Drop calories coming from fats and/or carbs by 250 calories per day (10g of fat + 40g of carbs = 250 calories).
- Add in one extra 20- or 40-minute cardio session per week.
- Make sure you're tracking your intake accurately.

Stress in general is the enemy when it comes to weight loss. So do anything you can to calm yourself down and lower your stress levels – listen to music, walk in nature, play with your dog, go to the cinema, anything that relaxes you.

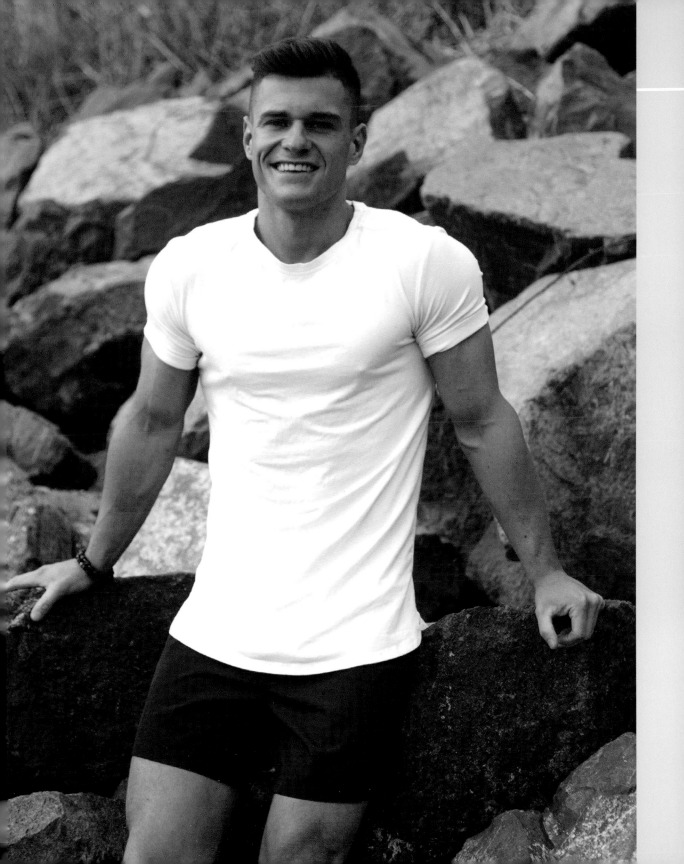

Micronutrients and fibre

We're all over *macronutrients* by now, but what about *micronutrients*?
Easy. Micronutrients are vitamins and minerals. These may not affect body composition directly or in the short term, but they do matter in the long term. If you end up with nutrient deficiencies, you'll get run down, sick, have poor health and become tired and drained. You can't train when you're sick, so this will massively impact your results. But don't worry, you don't have to track your micro intake the way you do your macros. There are vitamins and minerals in almost everything!

This is where a good dose of common sense comes in again. A Subway sandwich isn't as nutrient-dense as a large bowl of broccoli, but think about it: it still contains micronutrients and fibre from the lettuce, peppers, wholewheat bread, cucumbers, etc. Just because it's classed as 'fast food' doesn't mean it's devoid of nutrients.

So we've established that you don't need to track micronutrients, but there are some very simple guidelines you can follow to ensure that you're getting what you need.

"There are vitamins and minerals in almost everything!"

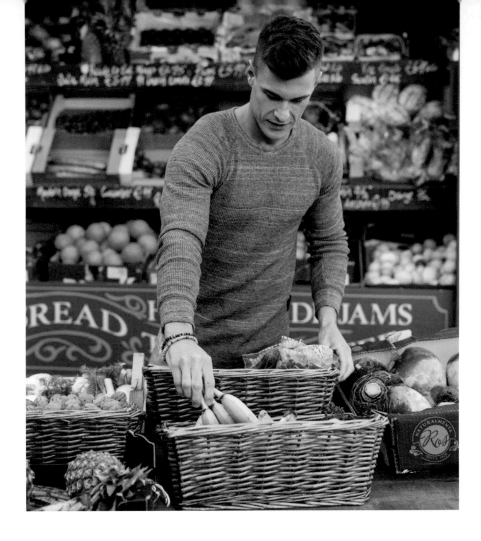

- Eat at least five servings of fruit and vegetables a day. An example of this could be two pieces of fruit a day (an apple and a banana) and three portions of veg (some broccoli, carrots and peppers).

- Eat fibrous vegetables with every meal. Add a side salad.

- Eat a *variety* of wholefoods, fruits and veg rather than the same things every day.

What counts as one portion of your five a day?

- 12 chunks of pineapple
- 8 Brussels sprouts
- 8 cauliflower florets
- 7 cherry tomatoes
- 3 stalks of celery
- 3 whole dried apricots
- 2 kiwi fruits
- 2 medium plums
- 2 small satsumas
- 2 broccoli florets
- 1 leek
- 1 medium apple
- 1 medium banana
- 1 medium onion
- 1 medium pear
- 1 slice of melon
- 1 handful of carrot or vegetable sticks
- ½ a large courgette
- ½ an avocado
- 3 heaped tablespoons of cooked kidney beans
- 3 heaped tablespoons of fresh or frozen peas
- 3 heaped tablespoons of tinned sweetcorn

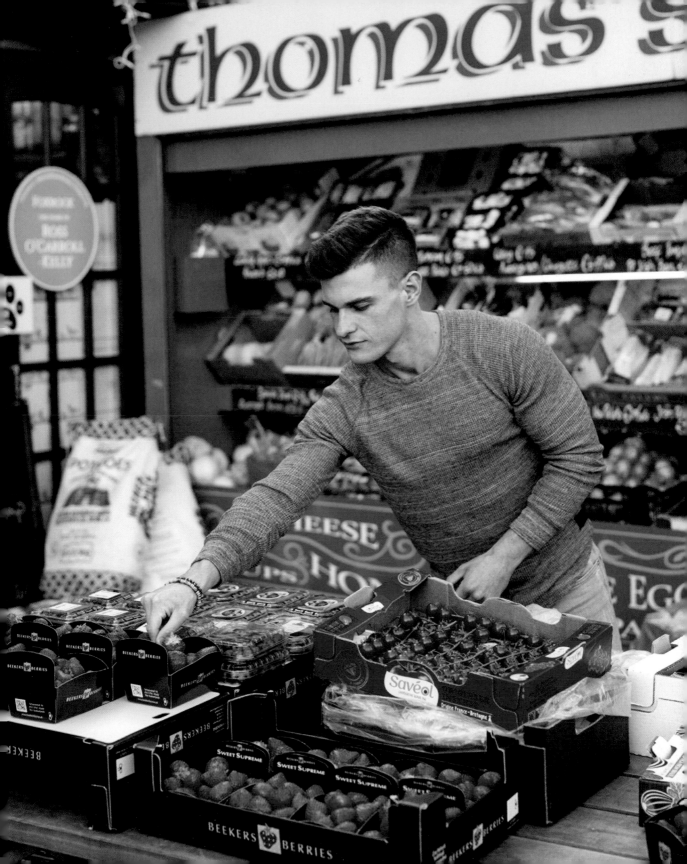

TAKE-HOME POINTS

> Eat five+ servings of fruit and/or veg every day.

> Eat plenty of high-fibre starchy carbs, such as:

- Apples
- Beans
- Berries
- Broccoli
- Brown rice
- Carrots
- Leafy greens, such as kale
- Lentils
- Mushrooms
- Potatoes
- Salads
- Squash

> Doing this will cover your micronutrient and fibre needs. One less thing to worry about!

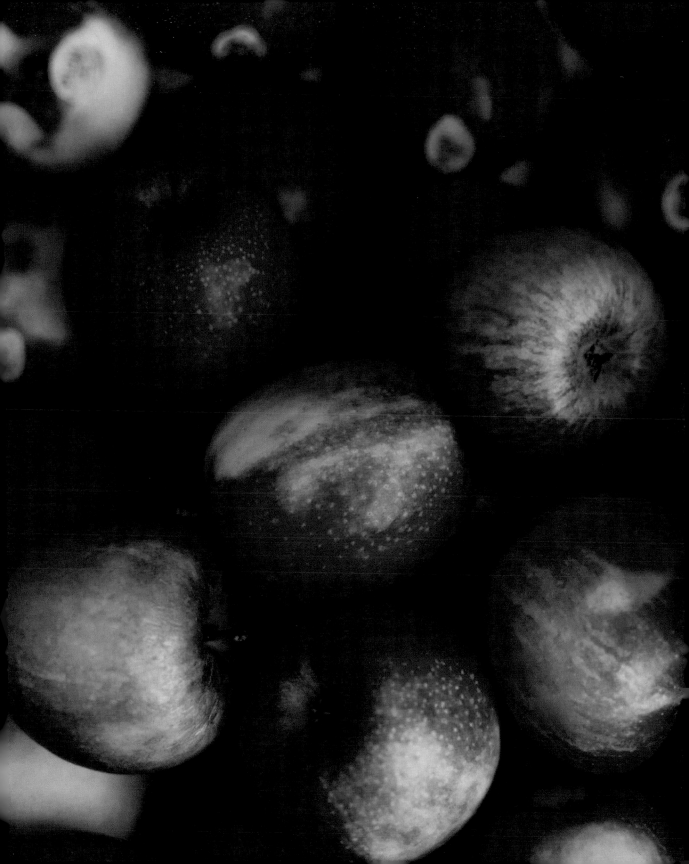

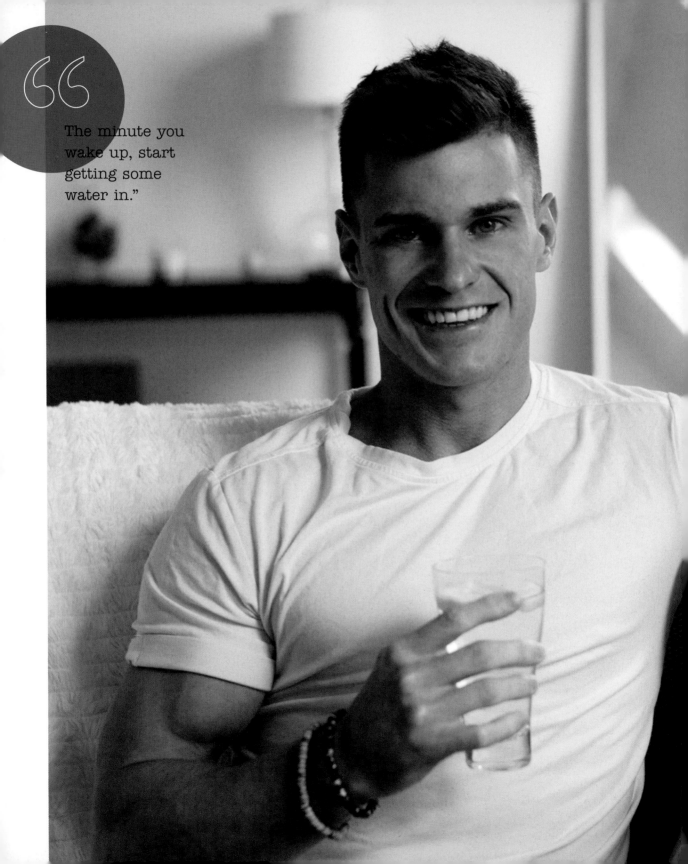

"The minute you wake up, start getting some water in."

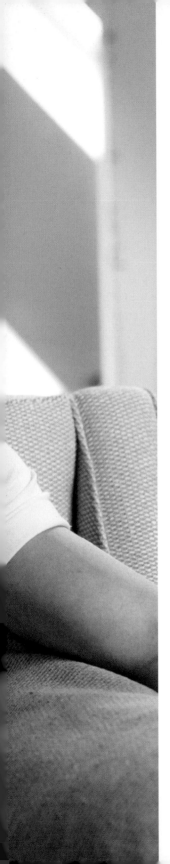

Keep hydrated

Many people overlook the importance of hydration. You've probably heard that the human body is approximately two-thirds water. However, this number barely begins to portray the importance of water from a muscle-building or training perspective. Dehydration has an incredibly negative impact on weightlifting as well as on muscular growth and recovery.

My advice for anyone regularly hitting the gym hard is to drink 3—5 litres of water a day. This isn't as hard as it sounds. For example, some of it will come from fruit, which is often 80 per cent water. You should also make sure you are well hydrated before training, so the minute you wake up, start getting some water in. This will also help with your cognitive function and focus.

As with micronutrients, the good news is that you don't need to track your water intake based on weight or anything like that — just make sure your urine is clear for the whole day. A tip for getting more water in is to add some zero-calorie or low-calorie flavourings to make it more interesting or add slices of lemon, lime or orange, some fresh mint leaves, some cucumber — whatever it takes to get it down you.

"We all know
the feeling
when we've
had a hard
day and turn
to comfort
food like pizza
and ice cream
to make us
feel better."

How to combat stress

It may not be as concrete as nutrition and training, but stress is a major problem to sort out if you want to see physical results. You can eat perfectly and train like a beast, but if your stress is at an all-time high, your progress will be seriously hampered.

I touched on this earlier, but let's now go further into the effect that stress has on fat loss and muscle gain. Since you need to eat more calories to gain fat, the stress hormone cortisol on its own isn't going to make you fat unless you're giving your body more energy than it burns. But stress and the resulting cortisol does affect appetite, which can of course result in weight gain. When the level of cortisol increases, so does appetite, in the form of cravings for high-carb, high-fat, high-sugar foods. We all know the feeling when we've had a hard day and turn to comfort food like pizza and ice cream to make us feel better. These foods are much easier to overeat than healthy foods. Added to this, when we're stressed or down about something we may start missing gym sessions or go in but not focus properly on having a good workout.

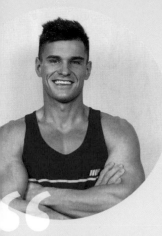

"Getting in a solid meal of protein, carbs and healthy fats first thing can set you up for a good day."

SO HOW CAN YOU COMBAT STRESS?

Clear your schedule
Use the time you've freed up to do something you find relaxing. Read a book, listen to music, go for a swim, walk your dog – it's up to you.

Exercise
Take your frustration out on the weights or even go for a vigorous hike, immersing all your senses in nature. Jump into the sea if you're near it.

Get enough sleep
I can't emphasize enough how important sleep is for recovery. Go to bed an hour earlier than usual, even if you still have work left to do. The work can wait till the morning. Aim for seven to ten hours a night, with eight being the ideal number. Some smartphones have a 'bedtime' function that will alert you when it's time to go to bed (you set up the ideal parameters yourself). Whatever it takes!

Don't turn to alcohol
A lot of people try to find relief from their stress by going out and having a few too many, but this just makes matters worse in the long run and burns a hole in your pocket. Alcohol is a depressant, so when you wake up the next day you'll feel even worse than before. The same goes for drugs.

Write it down
Plan out your days, and while you're at it, write down the things that are stressing you the most, then analyse the root of the problems and brainstorm how to solve them. Writing things down gets things out of your mind and on to paper, which can be very liberating. It also really helps with goal-setting.

Eat a good breakfast
If you have a crazy schedule, don't try to save time by skipping breakfast. Getting in a solid meal of protein, carbs and healthy fats first thing can set you up for a good day. Try some lean bacon, two whole eggs with two extra egg whites and some white potatoes.

Meditate
This is one of my favourite ways to bust stress, and it doesn't mean sitting on top of a mountain wearing a robe and going 'ohmmmmmm'. It can simply be making some alone time when you focus on your breathing and clear your mind of any negative thoughts.

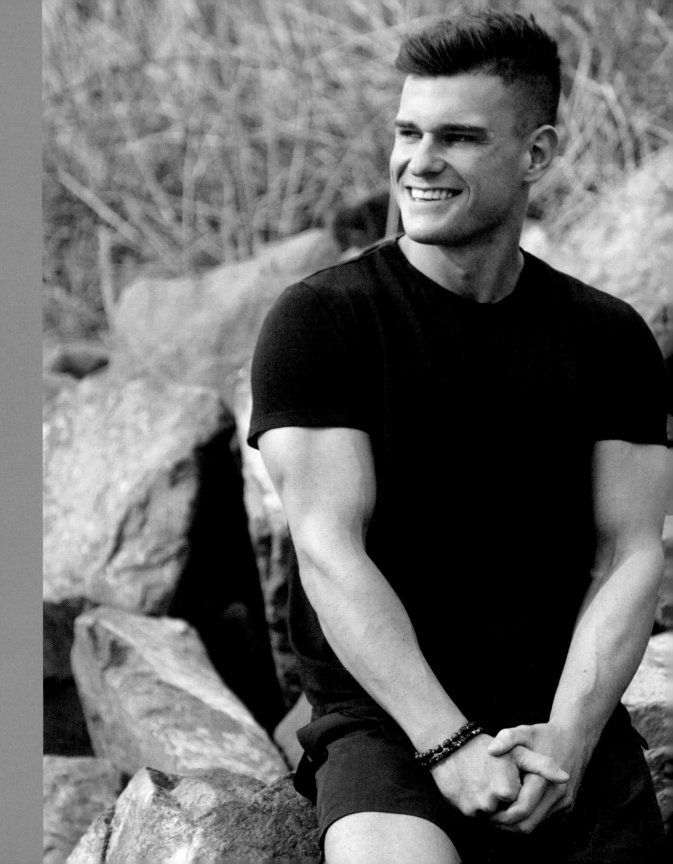

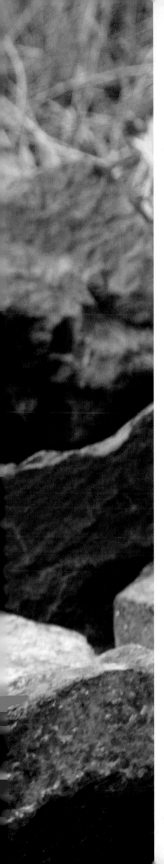

Nutrient timing

I know it sounds like I'm hitting you with science again, but nutrient timing is a very straightforward principle. Put simply, it refers to what you eat and when, in relation to exercise. It varies from person to person.

Nutrient timing is *not* important for:

- Weight loss or general health in overweight/obese people
- Fat loss or muscle gain in beginner/some intermediate trainees

Nutrient timing *might* be important for:

- Fat loss/muscle gain/strength gain in advanced trainees
- Intense training with fasting

Nutrient timing *is* important for:

- Athletes training more than once a day
- Athletes with intense events with little time between events
- Intense training/competitive events lasting more than two hours
- Anyone looking to get a small 1 per cent edge

1. HOW OFTEN SHOULD YOU EAT?

First things first: the 'eat little and often' advice has been relegated to the land of myths. The myth originally started with the TEF (thermic effect of food) principle. When we eat food, we use energy/calories to digest the food. It's easy to see why people thought that if you ate little and often you'd burn more calories, right?

The fact is that the TEF actually depends on the size of the meal/how many calories it contains.

So if you eat six meals with 500 calories each (3,000 calories in total) or three meals with 1,000 calories each (again, 3,000 calories in total), the TEF will be the same.

You can eat as many meals as you want to, but just make sure you're hitting your macros. The ideal would be three to four meals a day if you're looking to build some muscle (not one big meal a day, but I don't think anyone would want to do that anyway).

2. INTERMITTENT FASTING

Often shortened to IF, this practice involves skipping breakfast, narrowing your eating window down to eight hours a day and typically eating two large meals a day in that time. If you're used to eating breakfast (as most of us are), it will take at least a few days for your body to get used to the new meal pattern and for morning hunger pangs to decrease.

An example of a day of intermittent fasting could look like this:

- **8 a.m.**
  Wake up and have a black coffee or water (no calories) and go about your day. Coffee/caffeine can help a lot with hunger in the mornings. A zero-calorie energy drink is also a good option.

- **1–2 p.m.**
  Have your first meal of the day, for example a burrito bowl (see page 182).

- **5 p.m.**
  Have a small snack, such as an apple, some carrot sticks, my chocolate, chia and peanut butter protein balls (see page 194) or my chocolate and almond energy bites (see page 200).

- **9–10 p.m.**
  Have your last meal of the day, for example the creamy chicken, pea and pesto pasta salad on page 174.

TAKE-HOME POINTS

> As you are effectively skipping a meal when doing IF, the two meals you do have can be quite large and satisfying. You might not believe it, but if I'm doing IF, I can easily fit in a pizza (around 800 calories) every single day for dinner (I love pizza!). In general, getting to eat a meal you love every day can really help you to stick with the regime and give you something to look forward to.

> It seems counter-intuitive, but IF can help curb your appetite in the long run. Some breakfast eaters can find themselves getting hungry for a little snack with their coffee at around 11 a.m., but this will eventually stop happening when you skip breakfast.

> IF makes hitting your macros simpler. Remember, it all comes down to total macro intake, so if you eat fewer meals throughout the day, it will be easier to log and keep track of.

> Despite what your neighbourhood IF guru might try to sell you, I have to stress that intermittent fasting is not a magic spell that will instantly make you lean and toned. It still comes down to hitting your macros and being in a caloric deficit. Full stop.

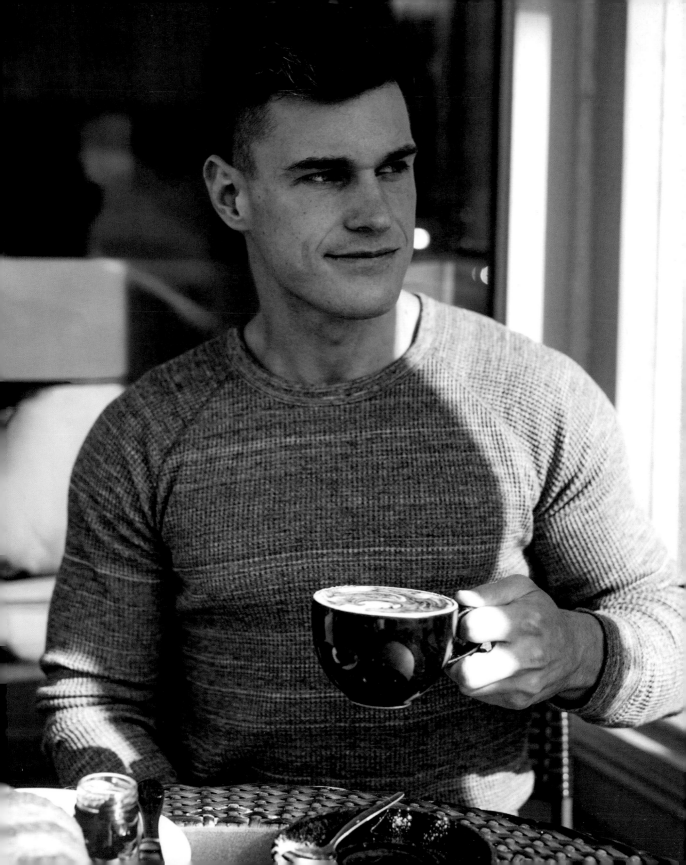

Carb backloading

Here's another scientific-sounding term that I'm going to take the mystery out of! Carb backloading basically combines intermittent fasting with eating regularly. I use this method myself when I'm preparing for a competition and trying to cut fat. Clients have had amazing results with this too.

So what exactly goes on when you're carb backloading? Put simply, you eat mainly protein (with some fats) during the day, saving most of your carb intake for the evening. An example of a day of carb backloading could look like this:

- **8 a.m.**
  Have a high-protein, low-carb, moderate-fat breakfast, such as my mini frittatas with bacon, spinach and cheddar (see page 165), a protein shake with almond milk and peanut butter or a high-fibre, low-carb protein bar.

- **1–2 p.m.**
  Have another high-protein, low-carb, low-fat meal, for example my Mexican chicken soup (see page 170).

- **5 p.m.**
  Post-workout, have your first meal with a high amount of carbs added in, such as the creamy chicken, pea and pesto pasta salad on page 174.

- **9 p.m.**
  Have your last meal of the day. This will be another high-carb, high-fat meal, such as my quick fish curry with basmati rice and broccoli (see page 192). Some people like this to be their highest-calorie meal so that they have something to look forward to at the end of the day.

TAKE-HOME POINTS

> When carb backloading, you still get to enjoy breakfast while building muscle mass, which is good for those who really dislike skipping breakfast.

> If you get late-night cravings, you can satisfy them with a large high-carb, high-fat meal.

> Some people get a 'brain fog' or feel lethargic after consuming a high amount of carbs in the morning. The high-protein breakfast won't do this and will leave you feeling sharper.

> Protein fills you up and stops you from getting hungry — it's satiating. Often when clients of mine have a high-protein breakfast they can go a long time without getting hungry or thinking about food.

> Carb backloading can help you sleep. A high-carb meal in the evening can release melatonin (a sleep hormone) in our bodies and make us drowsy, ensuring a good, deep sleep. As mentioned earlier (see page 81), sleep is a massive factor in body composition. For some reason oats make me sleepy, so I often have them before bed.

> You may be putting more effort into meal prepping, but it's unlikely that you'll lose muscle, which can be a danger with fasting.

> As with intermittent fasting, carb backloading isn't magic, so you need to stay on top of your macro intake.

Carb cycling and refeeds

This is another method that works by juggling your carb intake. Carb cycling has many different forms or approaches, so let's look at a few.

1. HIGH DAYS AND LOW DAYS

This means that you have a higher carb and lower fat intake on training days and vice versa on rest days. Some people really enjoy this approach and notice improved performance in the gym. However, I'm not convinced it works, plus changing your intake on a daily basis is unnecessarily complicated, especially for beginners who are new to tracking their intake and are trying to get a consistent eating pattern in place.

2. REFEED DAYS

I like this approach better and I believe it really works. Refeed days are essentially 'carbing up' and are added in for those on a dieting phase. They involve raising your carb intake 100 per cent while lowering protein and fat slightly. The lower your body-fat percentage is, the more frequently you should add a refeed day.

Here's an example of when you could add in a refeed day, related to your body-fat percentage.

- Over 20 per cent: No need for refeeds
- 15–20 per cent: Once every two to three weeks
- 10–15 per cent: Once every two weeks
- Under 10 per cent: Once a week
- Under 8 per cent: Twice a week

These are solid guidelines, but you should also add how you're feeling into the equation. If you're feeling depleted and weak in the gym, then it's probably time for a refeed. On the other hand, if you're full of energy and having great workouts, you don't need one. Keep pushing until you feel you really need a refeed day.

90

Here's a more concrete example of a refeed day. Say you're cutting calories and your usual intake looks like this:

- Protein: 200g
- Carbohydrates: 250g
- Fats: 50g

On a refeed day, it will look like this:

- Protein: 150g
- Carbohydrates: 500g
- Fats: 30g or less

It can be a challenge to take in 500g of carbohydrates while keeping fat intake low, so on the day eat lots of pasta, rice, cereal, jam, bananas, potatoes, sushi, oats, honey — anything high-carb and low-fat.

3. IS A REFEED DAY LIKE A CHEAT DAY?

The short answer is no. On a cheat day your fat intake, along with your calories, will skyrocket. In addition, cheat days are usually the result of an unplanned (quite often post-party!) binge. In contrast, a refeed day is taking place in a *controlled situation*. You're dropping your fat intake as low as possible and only increasing calories from carbs. In a person who has been dieting for a while, it's very difficult for carbs to be converted to fat.

TAKE-HOME POINTS

> Take the carb cycling/refeed approach you find easiest to follow.

> Your weekly macro/calorie average will still be the most defining factor.

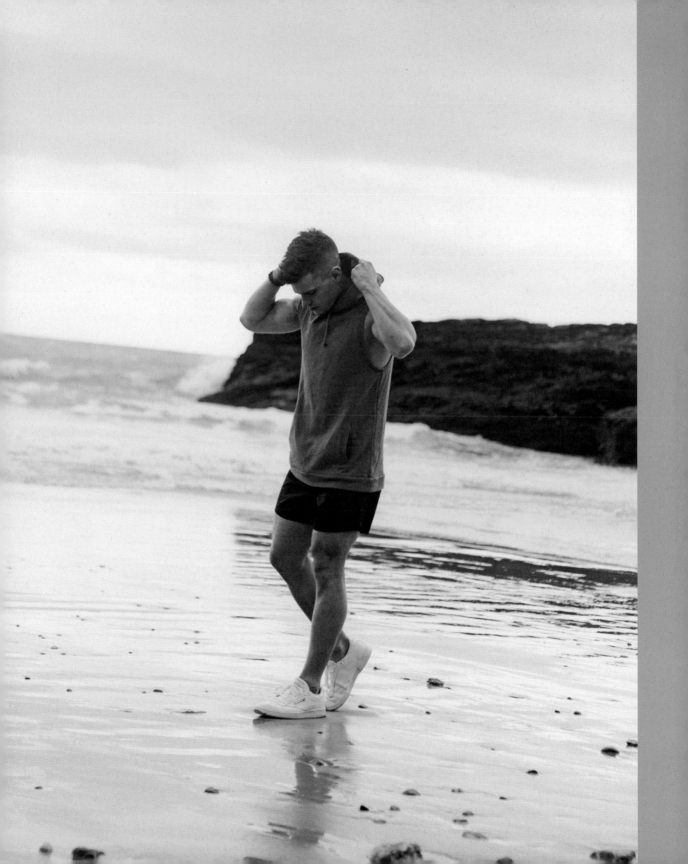

The full diet break

The mantra to remember for this method is one step back, two steps forward. As you may have guessed from the name, the full diet break is when you stop *dieting* for two to three weeks. This means that you go back to maintenance level on the calories (see page 42) and pull back on rigid tracking or hitting your macros to the gram. You increase your calories by raising your intake of carbs and fats.

"One step back, two steps forward."

HOW CAN THIS HELP?

As you know by now, dieting isn't a walk in the park and there are plenty of downsides. When losing weight, metabolism can slow down and food cravings can kick in. It's only human to struggle sometimes with the commitment and motivation – that's just part of dieting. Returning to maintenance for a few weeks is like pressing a reset button to return everything to baseline level. But don't worry, you're not bringing calories any higher than maintenance level, so you won't pile on the pounds.

Your performance in the gym will improve and your glycogen (a molecule in your body that stores your glucose fuel for later use) will be replenished. This should refresh you and remotivate you to go back on the dieting wagon once the break is done. Remember, one step back, two steps forward.

Cheat meals and untracked meals

There is really no such thing as a cheat meal. I'm actually not a fan of the phrase 'cheat meal' — putting the word 'cheat' in your diet adds a negative association to the meal, which can lead to unnecessary guilt and make people feel as if they've done something wrong. If you stay within your calories/macros but have a plate of pancakes on a Saturday, it's not a cheat meal.

A mate of mine, Ben Carpenter, uses a simple analogy to explain the concept of cheat meals while dieting. Let's say you want to save some money. You reckon you can save €350 per week, which averages out to €50 per day. On five days of the week you do really well and save €50 on each of them. On the other two days not only do you fail to save any money, but you go on a shopping spree and spend €100 on each of those days. So you save €250 over five days of the week but then spend €100 on each of the other two days. At the end of the week you only saved €50 instead of €350.

If someone asks you why you're struggling to save money, what do you say?

A	'The problem is that I need to save more during the week.'
B	'My savings account is broken.'
C	'My weekend habits damage the rest of my week's progress.'

Remember, you can call something a cheat meal, but it doesn't make the calories disappear. So many people say things like, 'I'm only eating X number of calories and I can't lose weight! I think I have a broken metabolism!' But after a few probing questions they'll admit that they eat three times as much as normal at the weekend.

I'm not against cheat meals per se. If you want to save up some calories and kick back with a pizza and a few beers on a Friday night, that's fine. Do what it takes to keep you sane and sticking to your diet for the most part. Just be aware of the net effect that this has over the course of the week. So the moral of the story is don't blame your savings account for being broken if you keep going on spending sprees.

BENEFITS OF CHEAT MEALS

Let's talk about factors that can be *beneficial* when it comes to cheat meals or untracked meals. A meal out or an untracked meal like a burger and fries is a great way to take the load off and let loose. In the long term, it can actually help you to stick to your diet as it makes it more bearable. On the day of the cheat meal (or even the day before if you know it's going to happen), do some extra cardio and reduce your carbs and fats slightly — we all know restaurant meals are often very high in carbs and fat/calories! That said, don't work out excessively or restrict your food intake too much, as this could lead to binge eating down the line. Just relax and enjoy your meal. If you follow the above guidelines, you'll most likely stay within or near your desired calorie goals.

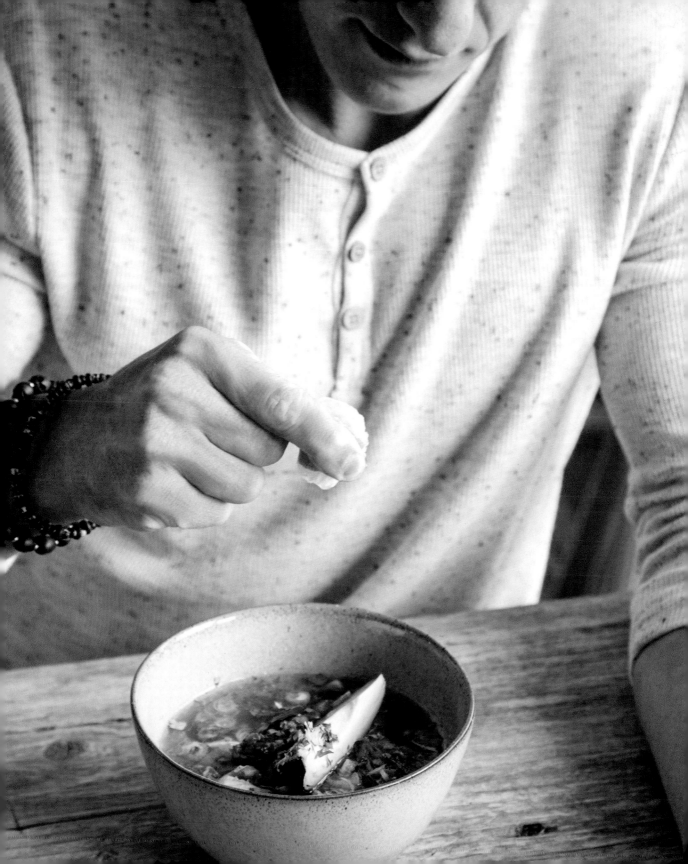

Peri-workout nutrition

Before you ask, this has nothing to do with what you order on your chicken at Nando's! It means what a person eats before (pre), during (intra) and after (post) training. The term 'peri' is a bit misleading, as it means 'about' or 'around' but not 'during'. Whatever it means, though, does it work magic? When I was younger I thought it did — I worshipped at the altar of protein powder, always carried a shake on me and even slept with a shake by my bed so I could get some quick gains in when I woke up! Let's go through the different elements of peri and see what it's all about.

1. POST-WORKOUT NUTRITION

This is by far the most talked about (and practised) of the three phases of peri-workout nutrition. Many people out there believe that you need to down a shake after your workout or else you'll miss the window of opportunity for those gains. Others think that you must refill your carb stores straight away or you'll never replenish the glycogen lost in a tough workout. I'm here to tell you that these are myths pedalled by biased supplement companies. Studies have shown that if you consume enough protein throughout the day, it's all good. The timing has nothing to do with it. Research has also shown that glycogen stores replenished themselves on the same day as a tough workout as long as total carbs were matched.

Let me give you some concrete examples, as I find they always make the science easier to understand. Say you do a daily workout at 1 p.m. and don't consume carbohydrates until 4 p.m. That's fine; your glycogen simply gets replenished then. The only people who need to think about replenishing glycogen stores are people who are training multiple times a day and need to be topped up for their next session. This would apply to a GAA, rugby or soccer player or an MMA fighter who has a conditioning session in the morning, then pitch/mat work in the evening. As you can see, for the majority of us, who just want to lose fat, build muscle and train once a day (or several times a week), this isn't a concern.

2. PRE-WORKOUT NUTRITION

Pre-workout nutrition is a different story. What you eat (or don't eat) before working out should enhance your performance in the gym or the field and allow you to perform at your best. As I'm always saying, trial and error are key here, as everybody is different, but the typical recommendation is to consume a decent amount of carbohydrates one to two hours before a session (20–25 per cent of your daily intake). Having said that, I have loads of clients who prefer to work out fasted, as they find that a carb-dense meal can make them feel lethargic. Others prefer to eat a light snack a few hours prior to working out.

3. INTRA-WORKOUT NUTRITION

This is really only for athletes engaging in two or more hours of *continuous* intense training. Something like a liquid carb source may come in handy if you have a weights session directly followed by a pitch session or conditioning. Intra-workout nutrition isn't necessary for most people. Okay, some of you may spend more than two hours in the gym (even though there's no real need to, in my opinion), but this includes a lot of resting and sitting around waiting for your next set, so it's not continuous exercise.

TAKE-HOME POINTS

> The most important thing is to take in your desired amount of calories, protein and carbs *by the end of the day*. Don't stress over what exactly you get before, during and after a workout. Keep in mind that it takes several hours to digest and fully absorb some nutrients, such as protein and fibre, so there is a constant overlap of nutrients being digested.

> Much of what you eat before, during and after working out will be determined mainly by personal preference, food tolerances and experience, and then by your athletic or bodybuilding goals.

> For pre-workout nutrition, use trial and error. Try a few different things that are easy to digest and find out what makes you feel your best and most energetic.

> There are no certain foods or amounts of foods that you have to eat before you hit the gym.

> Most of us don't need to even think about intra-workout nutrition — it's only for hardcore athletes.

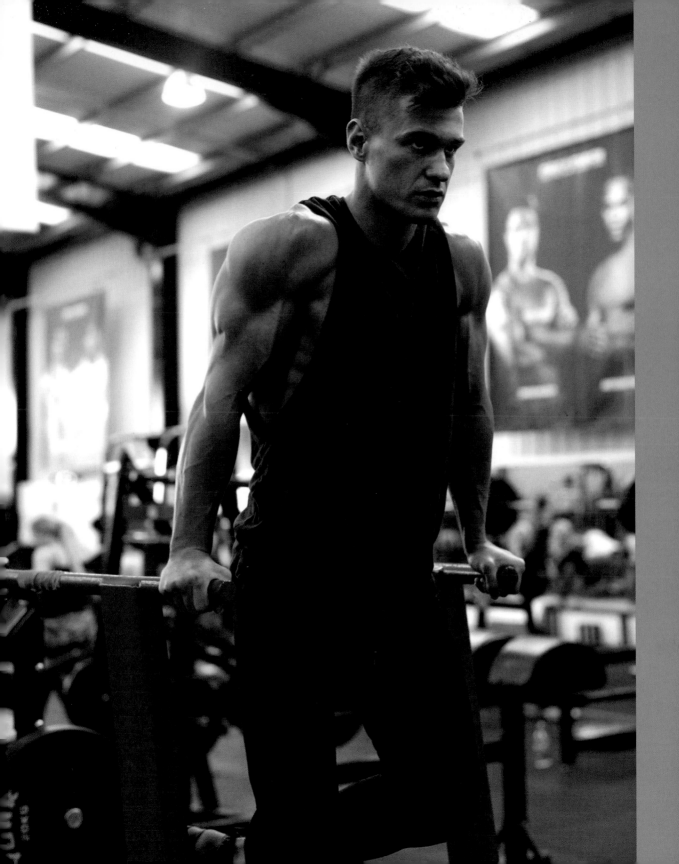

Supplements

It's just human nature that people will always look for the magic shortcut to avoid consistent hard work. This is where the world of supplements comes in. Don't get me wrong, they do have a place, but they will never be a replacement for solid hard work and consistent diet. Let's go through the main ones.

1. WHEY PROTEIN

Whey protein is a food source (technically, it's not a supplement) that is a by-product of dairy. It will allow you to hit your protein intake goals a lot more easily and also add variety and taste to your diet.

2. VITAMIN D

Vitamin D has a wide range of benefits, including increased cognition, immune-system health, bone health and general wellbeing. Taking a vitamin D supplement can reduce the risk of cancer, heart disease, depression, diabetes and multiple sclerosis. Most people don't get enough vitamin D, especially those of us who live in dark, cold countries, as you get it from sunlight. Research suggests that the true safe upper limit is 10,000 IU per day. For moderate supplementation, a 1,000–2,000 IU dose of vitamin D3 is sufficient to meet the needs of most of the population. This is the lowest effective dose range. Higher doses, based on body weight, are in the range of 20–80 IU per kg daily. Vitamin D should be taken daily with meals or a source of fat, like fish oil.

3. MAGNESIUM/ZMA

Magnesium is an essential dietary mineral and can become deficient when you are dieting/in a caloric deficit. If you're lacking in magnesium, you can get higher blood pressure and reduced glucose tolerance. It's best to take a magnesium supplement before bed, as it can improve sleep quality, which is also very important.

A ZMA supplement is even better, as it contains both zinc and magnesium. Zinc has many benefits, including boosting the immune system. The recommended dosage is roughly two capsules:

- Vitamin B6: 7mg
- Magnesium: 300mg
- Zinc: 20mg

4. CREATINE MONOHYDRATE

This organic acid occurs naturally in the body and helps to supply energy to all cells, primarily muscle. Despite what some people say about its side effects, taking a supplement can be worthwhile and will provide a host of health benefits. Taking 5g a day will help you to increase power output/ workload and therefore aid in building lean muscle.

5. FISH OIL

Fish oil is a type of fatty acid that comes from the tissues of oily fish, such as mackerel. It contains the omega-3 fatty acids, which provide multiple health benefits, including decreasing your risk of stroke and heart disease. A good dose to start with is 2–5g a day.

6. BETA-ALANINE (BA)

BA is often called the endurance version of creatine monohydrate. If you're in the bodybuilding world, it will help you do more reps and/or sets. BA can also help with high-intensity interval training (HIIT) cardio. An effective dosage is 3.5–5g a day.

7. BRANCH CHAIN AMINO ACIDS (BCAAs)

BCAAs are one of the most popular supplements out there, despite being one of the least effective. The fact is that if you regularly consume enough protein from different sources throughout the day you probably won't notice any benefit from these. I've taken BCAA supplements before and didn't notice a substantial difference. However, I have to say that some taste amazing and contain only a trace amount of calories, so I often use them to flavour water. To sum up, just buy high-protein food instead.

Socializing and alcohol

There is absolutely no point in training like a demon all the time if you have no life outside the weights room. You'll never stick to a training and nutrition plan anyway if you're not having any fun the rest of the time. So you've got a big night out on the horizon? Here are my top tips to get ready for it.

- Get in a good workout earlier that day and add in some extra cardio at the end so that you use up lots of energy/glycogen.

- Schedule your rest day for the day after.

- Avoid carb-laden drinks like beer and fruity stuff. Go for dry wines or spirits mixed with a zero-calorie soft drink (Monster Zero, 7 Up Free, etc.). I always go for vodka and a calorie-free energy drink.

- Lower the amount of fats you take in that day and don't eat any fatty foods, such as chips or crisps, while you're drinking.

- Get most of your calories that day from protein and some from carbs.

- Try to keep big nights out to every second weekend or, even better, once a month. Nights out will be more enjoyable and you will look forward to them more if you don't go out as often.

- Cook something healthy yet tasty earlier that day and put it in the fridge for when you come in that night. Try to avoid the greasy takeaway at the end of the night. Some options out there (think doner kebab and chips) are more than 3,000 calories – that could set you back an entire week of hard work!

- Drink as much water as possible before going to bed – I strongly recommend over a litre (you'll thank me in the morning!).

It's definitely possible to still get lean while consuming alcohol if you aren't getting blackout drunk. Check this out:

- 200ml of vodka = 320 calories
- 1g of carbohydrate = 4 calories
- 200ml of vodka = 80g carbs (320 divided by 4)

Let's say your daily carb intake was 200g. The day you wanted to consume your 200ml, you would just consume 80g carbs less (120g in total) and have your 200ml with a Monster Zero or Coke Zero. You could even consume 35g of fat (320 calories) less or a combination of both.

The only problem with this neat little sum is that one drink can lead to another, and another, plus a few pints and a takeaway at the end of the night and a hangover the next day where you just lie in bed all day feeling crap and skip the gym. But as long as you actually keep it to a few drinks, with low-calorie mixers, or light beers, it's all good.

All about abs

The question I'm asked most is, 'How do you get your abs to show?' The ab (abdominal muscle) obsession has been on the go for some time and people have been inundated with mad diets or regimes promising to banish belly fat forever. We get adverts popping up on the side of our internet browser with things like 'Try this one weird trick to burn belly fat!' or a TV commercial that promises to tone or sculpt a certain area on your body with some fancy machine.

> "When in a caloric deficit, fat loss will occur over the entire body."

The hard truth is that you cannot focus on a specific area (abs, triceps, lower back, inner thighs, etc.) with specific exercises to focus fat loss on that area. When in a caloric deficit, fat loss will occur over the entire body. Read that again and remember it.

Like it or not, we're all genetically predisposed to hold on to fat for longer in some places rather than others. Personally, my vulnerable fat-holding area is around my obliques. Does this mean I should do oblique crunches to burn fat off that area? Absolutely not. Keep cutting fat by remaining in a caloric deficit (see page 39) and it will all come off eventually. There are *no magic tricks*. If it was possible to reduce targeted areas of fat, you'd have people going around with ripped abs but fat faces and arms. How weird would that look?

Be aware that some people who are underweight will first need to gain muscle and build a foundation of strength through training before cutting down to build up not only their muscles around the midsection but the rest of their body too. With that in mind, let's move on to the training section of this book to get those workouts going!

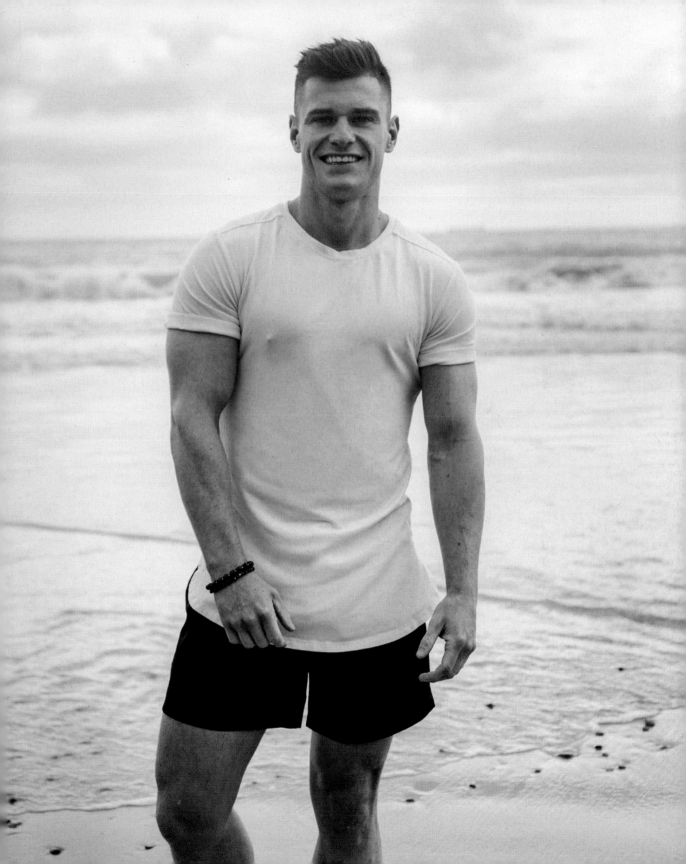

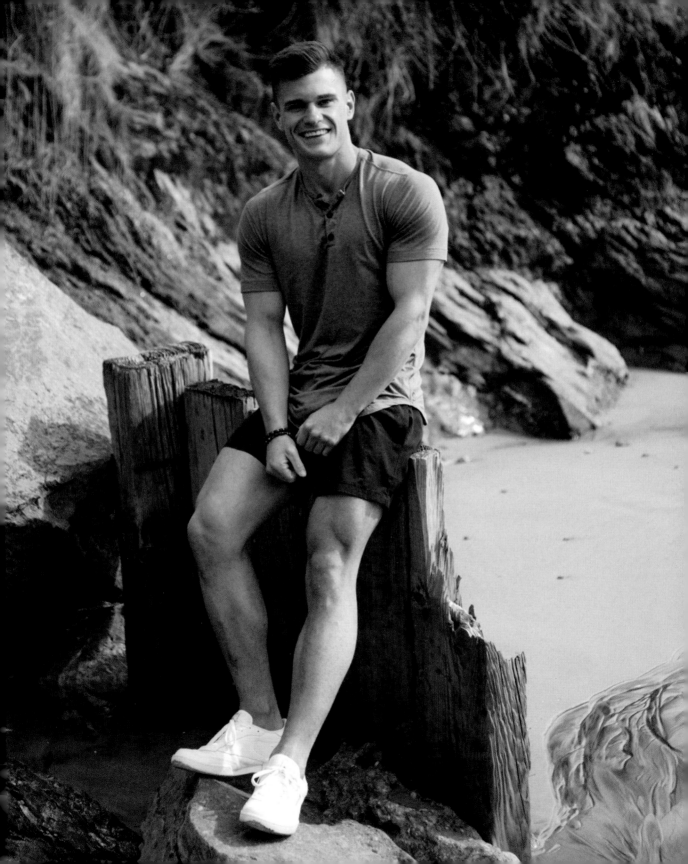

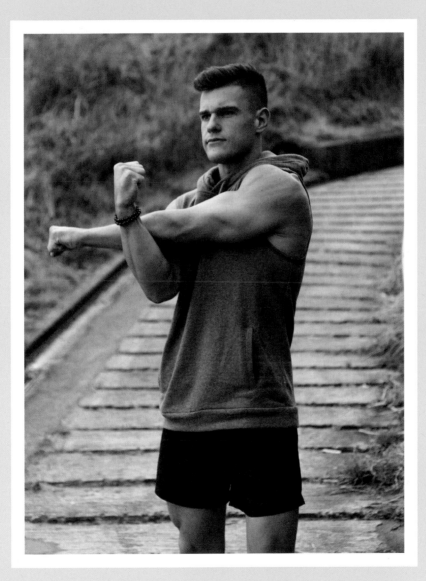

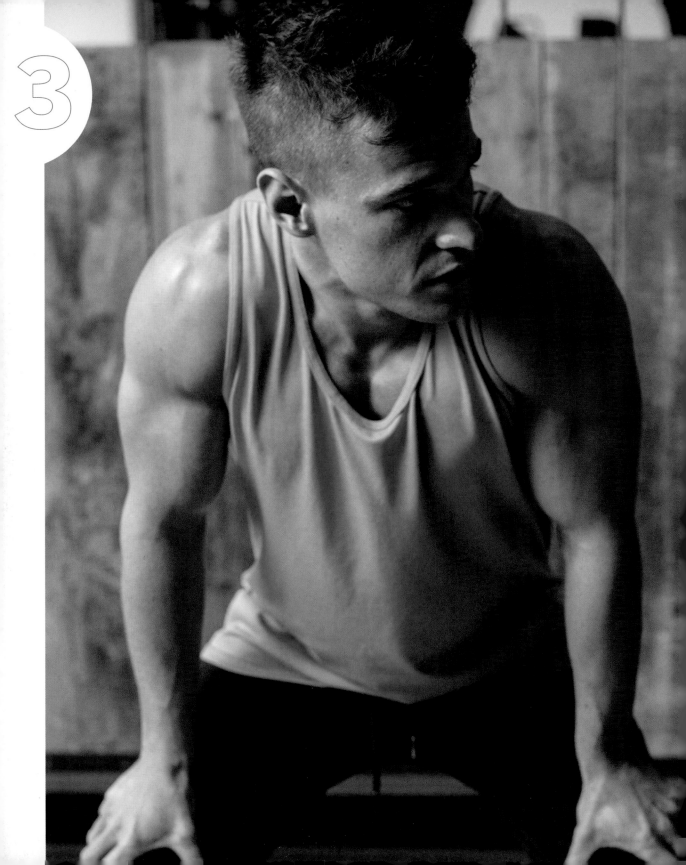

THE
TRAINING
PLAN

So we've killed the nutrition part, but if you want to gain muscle, strength and fitness, you need to combine your good nutrition with a regular training programme. You'd laugh if you saw the first training programme I put together for myself years ago when I was just getting started in the gym (but you'll never see it — I burned it!). I put it together from a combination of bodybuilder magazines and random things the super-buff guy in the changing rooms told me. There was no thought given to a balanced workout — I just set aside a day for each muscle: biceps day, triceps day, quad day . . . you get the idea. In those uninformed days, I believed that I had to let a body part rest for a week before I could train it again. I hated it! Imagine you loved bench pressing but thought you could only do it once a week!

Note:

I want to address an important point to dispel any confusion before we go any further. Some of my clients ask me, 'Can I gain muscle at the same time as losing body fat?' The short answer is yes, but only in some highly specific scenarios. For most people, it's unrealistic to aim for muscle gains and fat loss at the same time. Those who try usually end up spinning their wheels and making no progress. The exception is the person who has a high body-fat percentage and hasn't trained consistently before adopting a structured programme. To really simplify things, body fat is stored energy (calories = energy), so an overweight person has plenty of energy to pull from. Also, if you're new to training, you make more progress at the beginning due to the new stimulus you're providing, plus it's easier to add weight to your lifts. Combine this with a slight caloric deficit (see page 39), good sleep/ recovery and plenty of protein, and you will build muscle by increasing the weight you're lifting and lose body fat due to being in a caloric deficit. It's a rare scenario, though, and genetics will also play a big role.

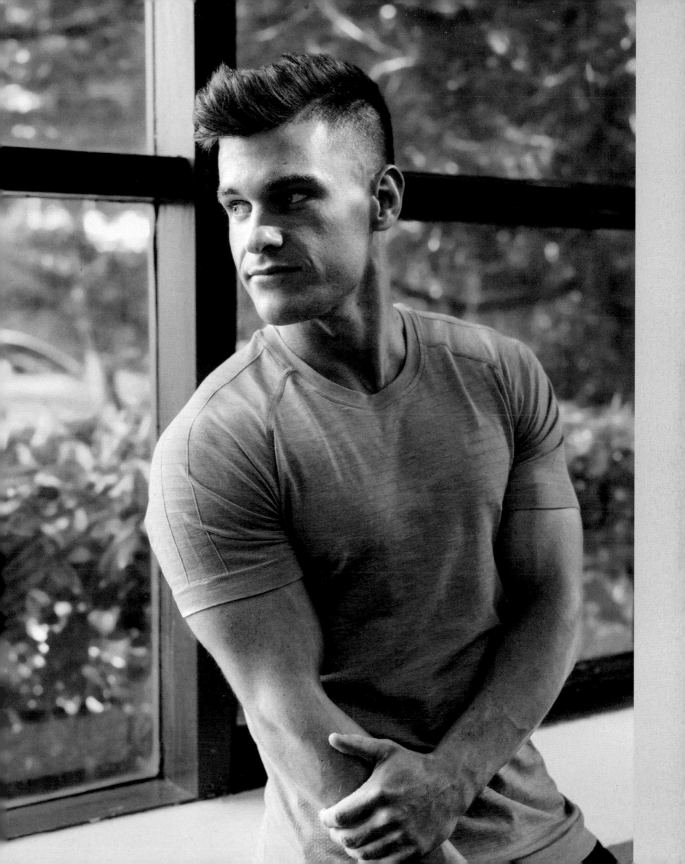

Enjoy your gym time

You have to consider a lot of factors that have nothing to do with training when planning your programme. After all, what's the point if you're stressing yourself out trying to fit in training? Stress is the enemy of losing body fat (see page 80). For example, if you're doing a demanding college course and working a part-time job in the evenings or if you have young children with limited childcare, you're simply not going to be able to make it to the gym five days a week. It's just not realistic. The key is to plan a programme that takes your schedule and lifestyle into account so that you aren't tying yourself in knots trying to attain something that's impossible.

Another important point to mention is to be sure to include lots of exercises that you love to do, which means that you'll be looking forward to sessions instead of dreading them! This will help you to stick to your programme, stay motivated and, most importantly, achieve results. It will then become like a sweet cycle, because seeing progress will motivate you to keep training.

Frequency and recovery

Frequency simply refers to the number of times a week you go to the gym or how many times you target a muscle group. It's really, really important to spread your training properly over the week. Doing a killer sesh on legs one day in a whole week isn't going to cut it, nor is doing a killer sesh seven days a week with no rest days. Neither option allows for recovery through proper sleep, nutrition and rest between sessions. Think of it this way (get ready for one of my analogies): say you're doing sunbed sessions to get a tan (I know, I know, no one in their right mind does this any more, but it's just an analogy!). You can do 5 minutes per session and distribute this across three sessions throughout the week to leave you with a nice golden tan or you can do 15 minutes in one session and end up with a nasty sunburn. The ideal target to aim for when you start out is three days a week, with the other days of the week being rest days to allow your muscles to recover (and grow), while maybe doing some gentle stuff like walking (see the section on NEAT on page 67 for more on this).

> "The key is to plan a programme that takes your schedule and lifestyle into account."

The whole point of training is to enhance your life, improve your mindset and enjoy the fruits of your labour in the form of improved posture and physique. Overtraining must be avoided, as progress will be difficult. Let me explain this with yet another analogy: imagine a sink with the tap running. The water flowing in is the exercise you're doing (this can also be applied to stress). If you're doing it at a reasonable rate, leaving enough recovery time so that you can train better next time, then happy days, the water will flow down the drain and everything will be good to go. But if you overdo it and put yourself under too much pressure, the water will build up and overflow.

> It's really, really important to spread out your training properly over the week."

Setting up your training

Let me start off by explaining how lean muscle mass is built, since this is what we're all aiming for in this process, to varying degrees. The fact is that nothing is going to work better to get this result than weight training. When you lift weights, the muscles you're using to do so get a bit damaged and torn. This doesn't sound good, but our bodies are designed to cope with this by rebuilding and repairing the muscles after your session. Eating the proper foods and amounts (see the Nutrition and Recipe chapters) contributes to this repair. The result? More defined and bigger muscles. Don't worry, weight training won't make you look like a bodybuilder if you don't want to. You control the process, so you can aim towards lean definition or adding noticeable mass if you choose to. Once you're on the journey, you can build up the weights over time as you feel able. It's also important to combine weight training with some cardio work, which I recommend doing two to three times a week. But more on that later (see page 143) — let's get started on the workouts.

I've included three of my favourite workouts: one for beginners, one for intermediate gym users and one for advanced gym users. You'll be able to do some of the bodyweight exercises at home (especially if you're a beginner and haven't found a gym yet), but most will need you to visit your local gym and use the weights they have there.

A FEW THINGS TO KEEP IN MIND...

1. Do some warm-up exercises to get your blood flowing before you hit the weights. These can include jogging on the spot, bodyweight squats, press-ups or shoulder rotating (see page 146).

2. If you're a complete beginner, you can try doing bodyweight exercises. This also applies to using some of the equipment in the gym – for example, an absolute beginner might start off doing squats with just the bar (i.e., no added weights on it).

3. Pick a weight you can do eight to ten reps of with proper form. If you're struggling or if your form is all out of whack, you've aimed too high with the weight.

4. Rest between each set for at least 1 minute or as long as it takes until you feel able to do the next set. You don't need to have a timer for this, just gauge how you feel.

5. You can substitute one exercise for another as long as the movement is more or less the same. So if you're deciding between a dumbbell bench press and a barbell bench press, go with the one you like best. The better choice will always be the one you prefer and feel more comfortable doing. Remember, just like a diet, you've got to like your training plan in order to stick to it.

6. If you're in doubt about anything you're doing or if something doesn't feel right or is causing you pain while you're at the gym, don't hesitate to ask for advice from one of the trainers. That's what they're there for.

Okay, let's do this!"

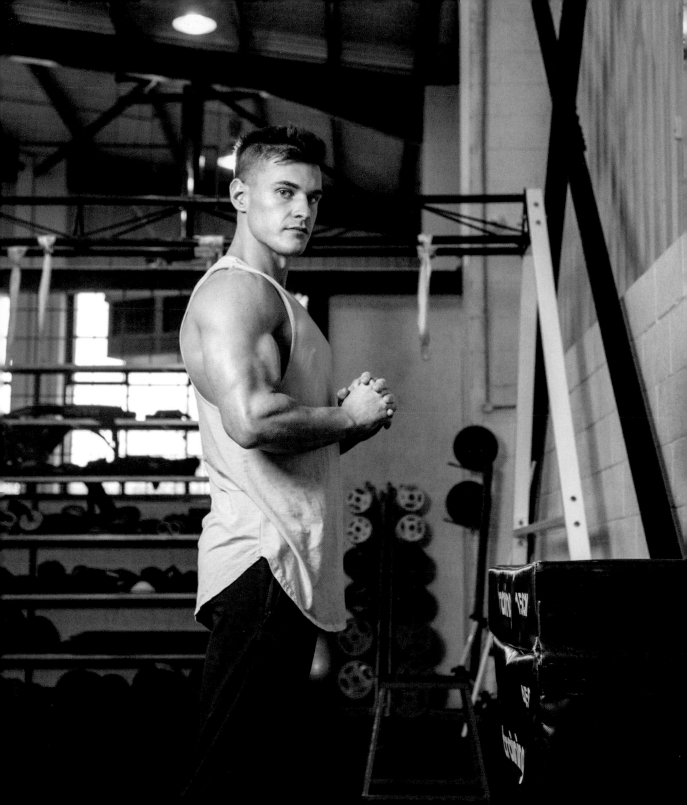

GLOSSARY OF **BASIC TRAINING TERMS**

- **AMRAP:** As many reps as possible.

- **COMPOUND EXERCISES**: These are the type of exercises that work more than one muscle at a time. They include squats, lunges and deadlifts.

- **DROP SET:** This applies to people who are at an intermediate or advanced stage in their training. Once you've finished a set of a certain exercise (for example, a bench press), drop (reduce) the weight and continue with a few more reps until you can't do any more. This allows you to get more work done in a shorter time period.

- **FORM**: The way in which you carry out your exercises. You should only lift weights that you are able to lift with the correct form, i.e., with good posture and no swinging.

- **ISOLATION EXERCISES**: These work just one muscle, for example a tricep curl.

- **REPS**: Short for repetitions. This refers to the number of times you do an exercise. For example, if you're given ten reps on a shoulder press, you do it ten times.

- **SETS**: This refers to how many times you repeat a given number of reps. For example, if you have to do three sets of eight reps on a back squat, you repeat the eight reps three times, with a rest between each set.

- **SUPER SET**: In a super set, you combine two or more different exercises within a set, such as a back squat and a back lunge.

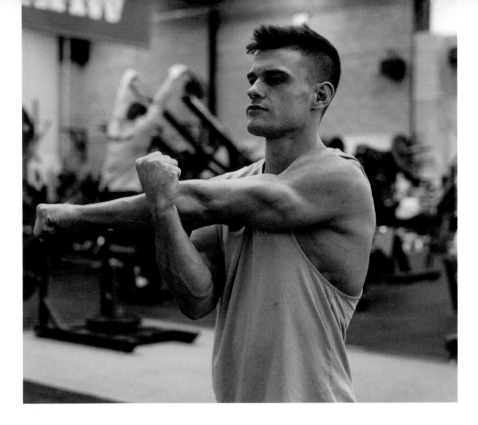

> "The more you look forward to something, the more likely it is that you're going to do it, and do it well."

Note:

I've allowed for rest days in all of these plans, so for the beginner plan a week looks like this:

- **DAY ONE:** Training
- **DAY TWO:** Rest
- **DAY THREE:** Training
- **DAY FOUR:** Rest
- **DAY FIVE:** Training
- **DAY SIX:** Rest
- **DAY SEVEN:** Rest

As you move up to intermediate and advanced plans, the number of rest days per week decreases.

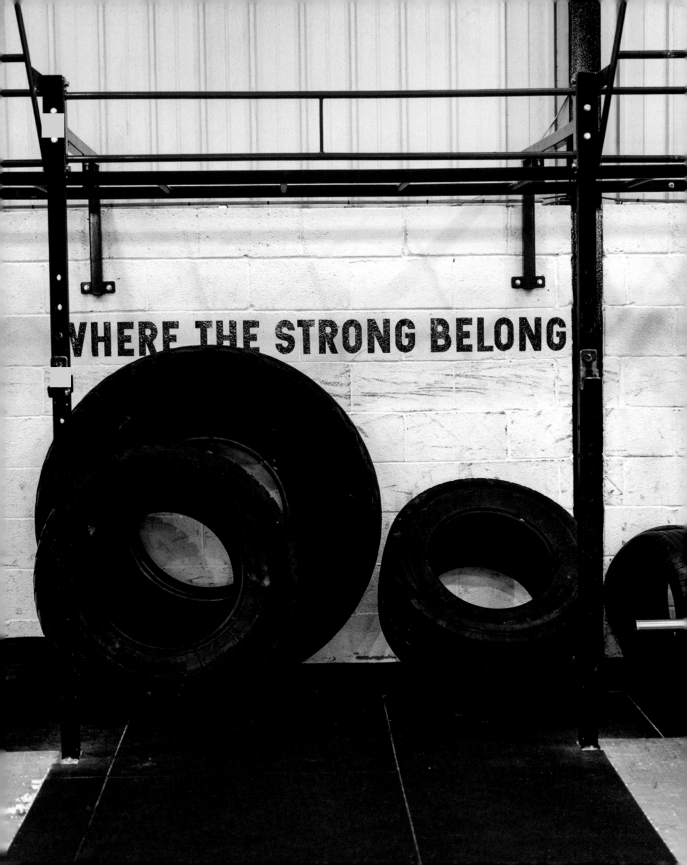

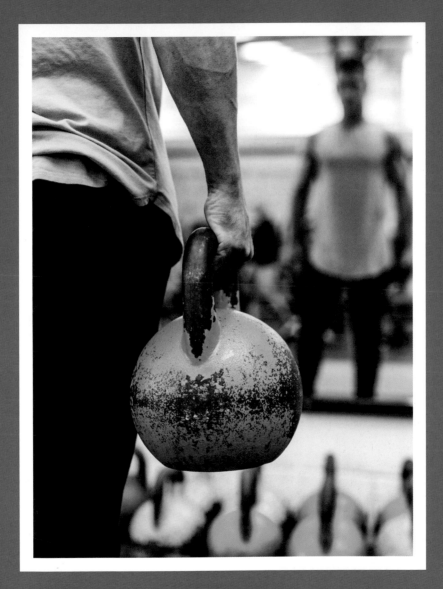

TRAINING PLAN 1:

BEGINNERS — THREE-DAY FULL BODY

DAY ONE: Full Body A (*Squat Focus*)

Exercise	Sets	Reps
Back squats (or bodyweight squats if you are a complete beginner)	3	8
Bench press	3	10
Barbell rows	3	10
Alternating bicep curls	3	10
Chest flyes	3	10
Triceps pushdowns	3	12

DAY TWO: Rest

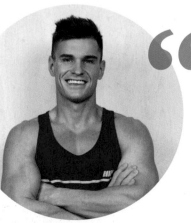

"The whole point of training is to enhance your life, improve your mindset and enjoy the fruits of your labour in the form of improved posture and physique."

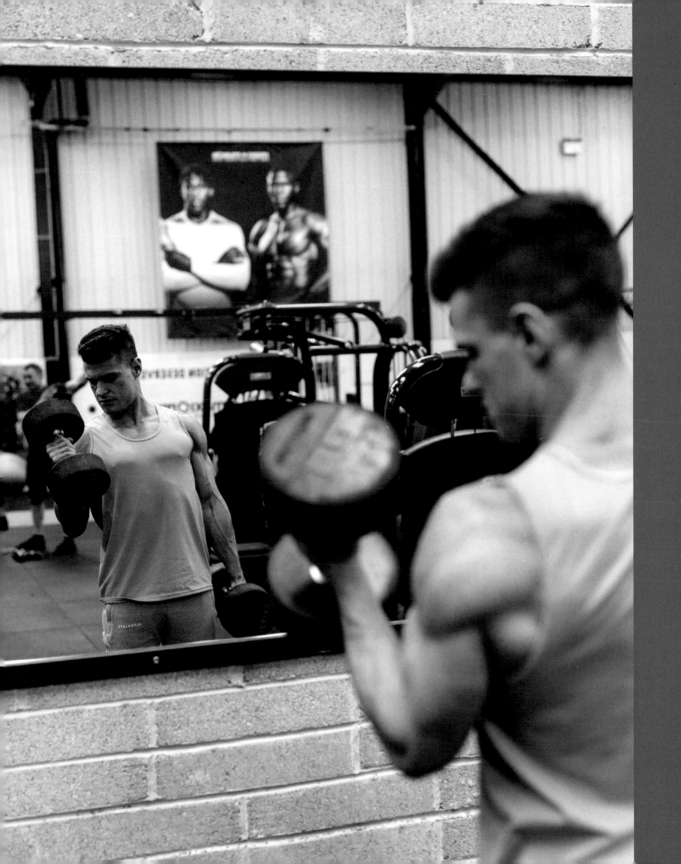

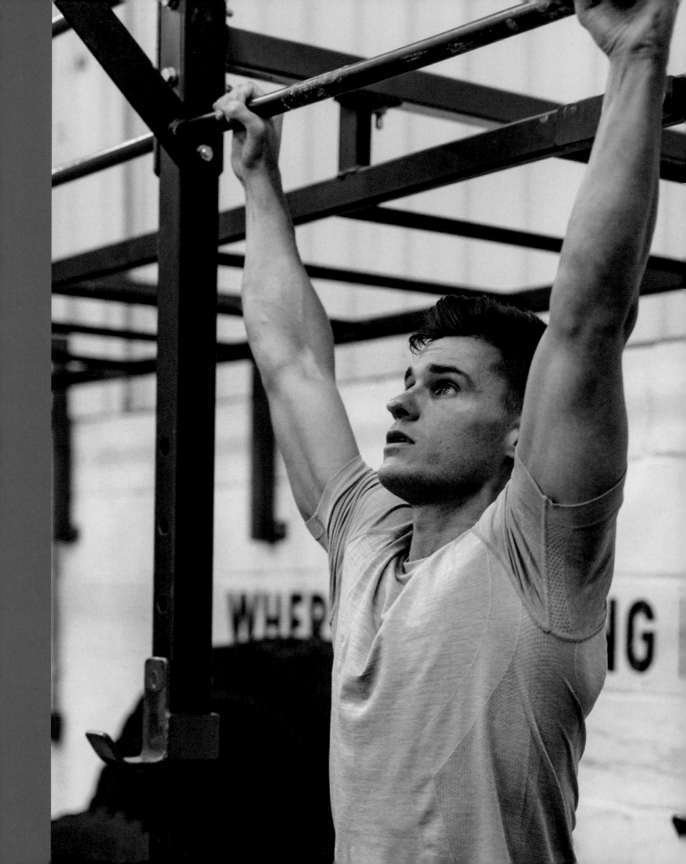

DAY THREE: Full Body B (*Bench Focus*)

Exercise	Sets	Reps
Flat bench press	3	8
Barbell squat	3	10
Incline dumbell press (*very slight incline*)	3	10
Shoulder press	3	10
One-arm rows	3	10 per arm
Triceps dumbbell kickbacks	3	10

DAY FOUR: Rest

DAY FIVE: Full Body C (*Deadlift Focus*)

Exercise	Sets	Reps
Straight leg deadlifts	3	8
Assisted pull-ups	3	8
Barbell squats	3	10
Flat dumbbell presses	3	10
Walking lunges	3	15 per leg
Abdominal crunches	3	20

DAYS SIX & SEVEN: Rest

TRAINING PLAN 2:

INTERMEDIATE — FOUR-DAY UPPER & LOWER BODY

DAY ONE: Full Body A (*Squat Focus*)

Exercise	Sets	Reps
Incline bench press	3	8 (drop set on the last set)
Assisted flat dumbbell presses	3	8
Upright rows	3	10
Chest flyes	3	10
Lateral side raises	3	10 (drop set on the last set)
Overhead tricep extensions	3	10
Bicep preacher curls	3	12

Day Two: Lower Day A (*Legs & Core*)

Exercise	Sets	Reps
Back squats (aim for depth)	3	8 (drop set on the last set)
Straight leg deadlifts	3	8 (drop set on the last set)
Calf raises	3	15
Abdominal crunches	3	20
Weighted planks	3	One-minute holds

Day Three: Rest

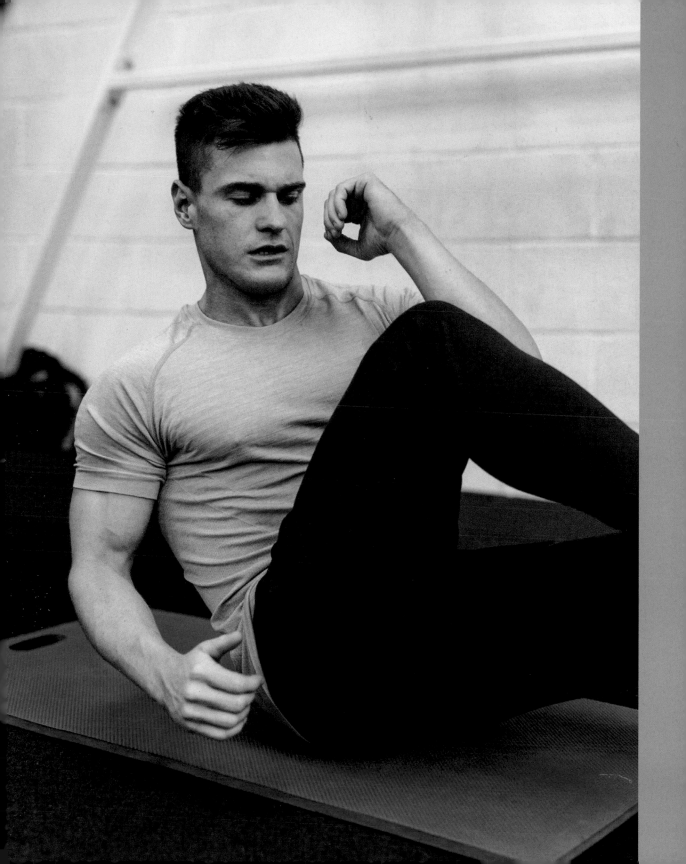

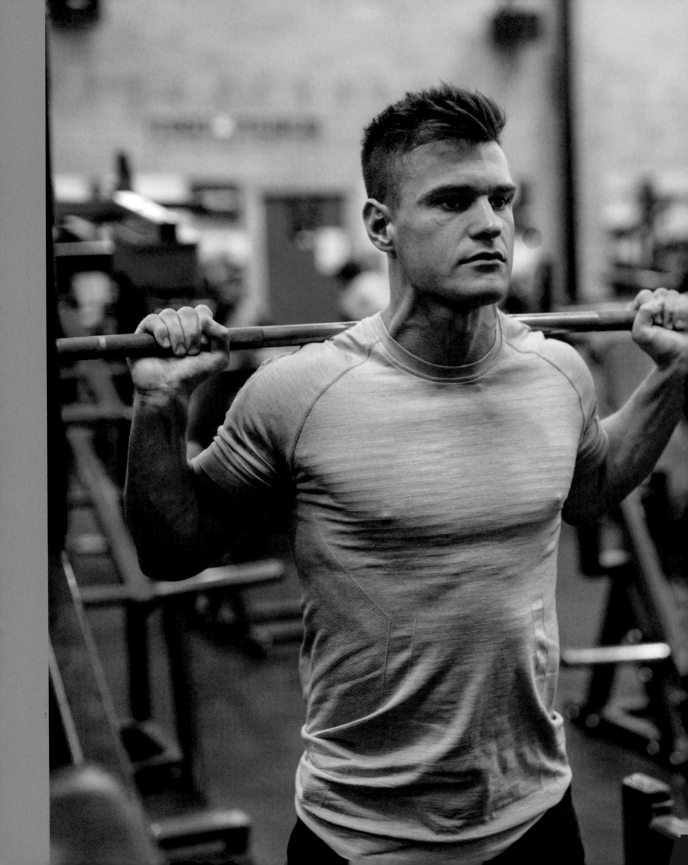

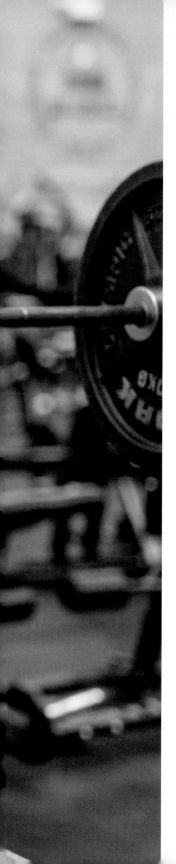

Day Four: Full Body B (*Bench Focus*)

Exercise	Sets	Reps
Assisted pull-ups (with a band)	3	8 (drop set on the last set)
Incline bench presses	3	8 (drop set on the last set)
Barbell rows	3	8
Lateral side raises	3	8
Banded face pull	3	10
Standing alternating dumbbell curls	4	10
Tricep pushdowns (with a machine or a band)	4	10

Day Five: Full Body C (*Deadlift Focus*)

Exercise	Sets	Reps
Straight leg deadlifts	3	8
Back squats	3	8 (drop set on the last set)
Calf raises	3	8
Weighted crunches	3	8
Planks	3	One-minute hold

DAYS SIX & SEVEN: Rest

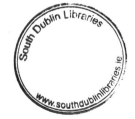

TRAINING PLAN 3:

ADVANCED — FIVE-DAY LEGS/PUSH/PULL/ UPPER & LOWER BODY

DAY ONE: Legs & Abdominals

Exercise	Sets	Reps
Back squats	3	8 (drop set on the last set)
Straight leg deadlifts	3	8
Leg extensions	3	10
Hamstring curls	3	10
Calf raises	3	15
Weighted decline crunches	3	20
Weighted planks	3	One-minute holds
Cable crunches	3	15

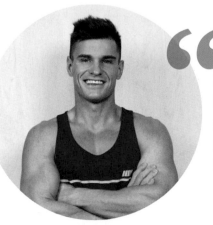

"If you tell me you don't need more than five hours of sleep a night and don't eat enough calories and no carbs, I don't expect your training to be very successful."

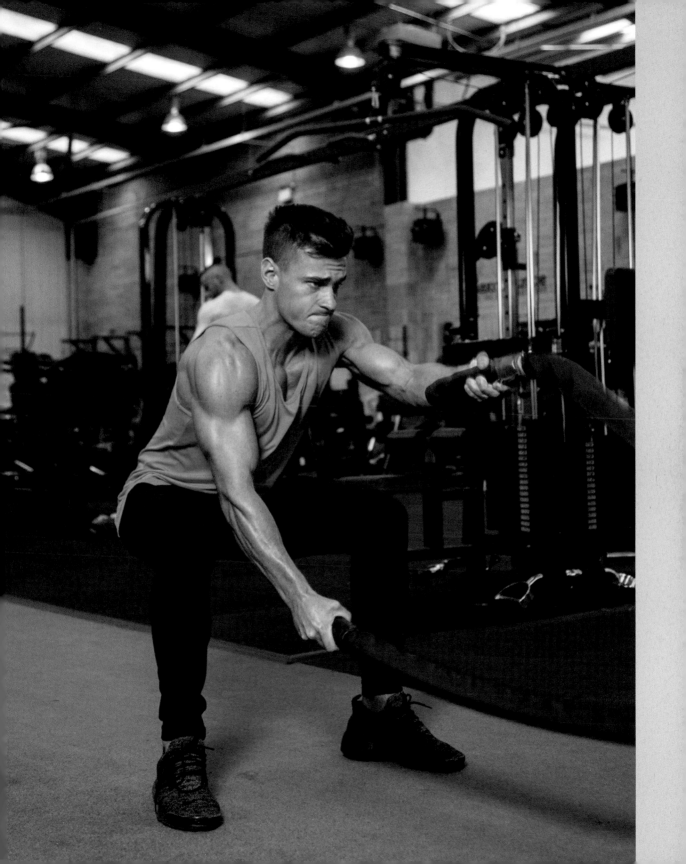

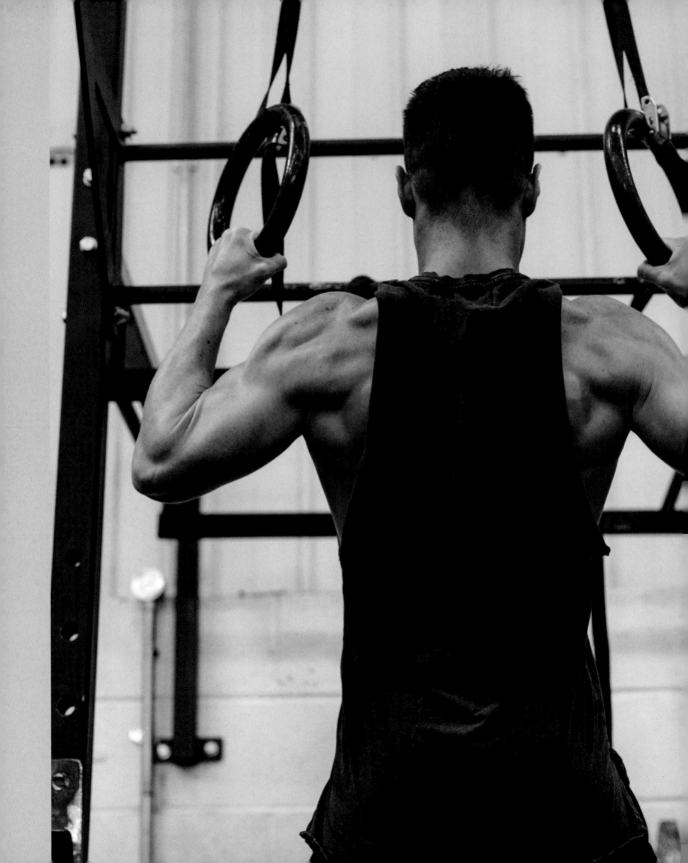

DAY TWO: Push Day (*Chest Focus*)

Exercise	Sets	Reps
Flat dumbbell presses	3	8 (drop set on the last set)
Incline machine presses	3	8
Dumbbell shoulder presses	3	12
Lateral side raises	3	12
Rear delt flyes	4	10
Cable chest flyes	4	10–12
Tricep pushdowns	3	10–12
Overhead tricep extensions	3	10–12

DAY THREE: Pull Day

Exercise	Sets	Reps
Narrow-grip pushdowns	3	8
Barbell rows	3	8
Wide-grip lateral pulldowns	3	8
Straight bar curls	3	10
Dumbbell curls	4	10
Hammer curls	3	10
Dumbbell shrugs	3	10
Bent-over one-arm rows	3	10

DAY FOUR: Rest

DAY FIVE: Upper Day (*Chest Focus*)

Exercise	Sets	Reps
Incline paused bench presses (bar to chest, slight pause before lifting)	3	8 (drop set on the last set)
Lateral pulldowns/weighted pull-ups	3	8
Flat dumbbell presses	3	10
Cable/banded face pulls	3	10
Cable chest flyes	3	10
Tricep pushdowns	3	10
Barbell curls	3	10

DAY SIX: Lower Day (*Legs & Core*)

Exercise	Sets	Reps
Deep back squats (if you're finding it hard to get the depth, replace with goblet squats)	3	8 (drop set on the last set)
Deadlifts	3	8
Leg extensions	3	10
Hamstring curls	3	10
Calf raises	3	12
Weighted decline crunches	3	20
Weighted planks	3	One-minute holds

DAY SEVEN: Rest

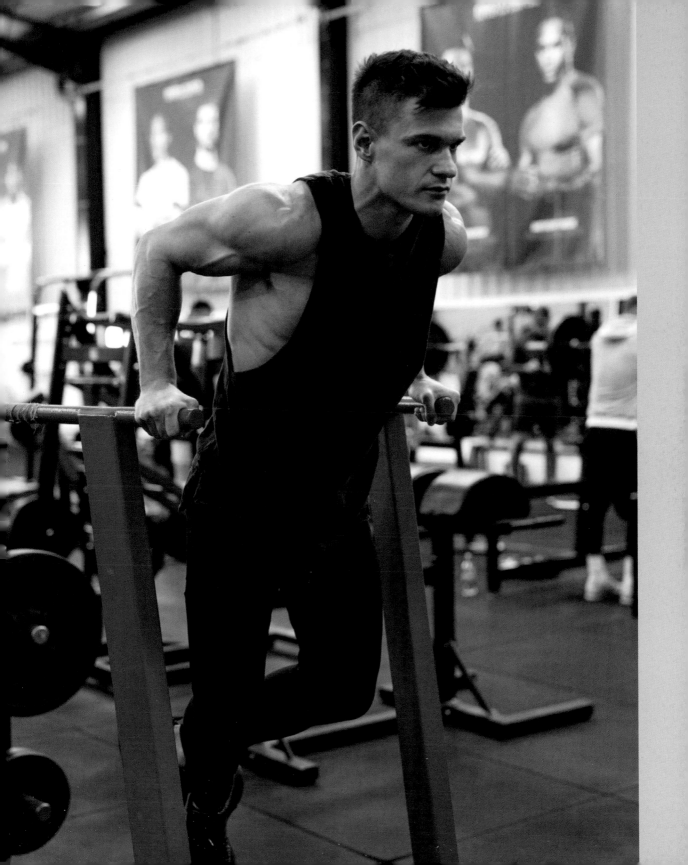

Troubleshooting the workouts

So you've had a chance to look at my proposed workouts but may be wondering which one to choose. Don't be misled into thinking that if you want to get into shape ASAP you need to go straight for the five-day plan. This may not be the case. You don't want to go from nothing to five days a week — instead, you want to build up your training regime or workload over time (remember my sunbed analogy!). I'd advise a beginner to follow the three-day programme as given until you feel you can increase the weight a bit and are used to performing the exercises correctly, tweaking it yourself to see what feels right while never compromising form.

What if you've been following a training plan for a while and you notice you're not making progress, either in strength or muscle gain? You've hit a plateau — a stall in your progress. The truth is that you're likely to progress at a more tangible rate if you're coming from no training than if you're a seasoned gym user. Progress isn't a straight line and a plateau for a beginner will be very different from a plateau for someone who is an advanced trainee. So before you throw your gym gear and new water bottle out of the pram, ask yourself a couple of questions:

> "Progress isn't a straight line and a plateau for a beginner will be very different from a plateau for someone who is an advanced trainee."

- **ARE YOU EATING ENOUGH?** You can't expect to keep lifting heavier weights without taking in more calories to compensate for it. You may be desperate to lose fat, but a few lettuce leaves and pumpkin seeds aren't going to cut it when you're working your body like that. See the Nutrition chapter for more on what you should be eating when in a training regime.

- **ARE YOU GETTING ENOUGH SLEEP?** This is non-negotiable. Sleep supports so many things, from muscle gain and fat loss to diet adherence, cognitive function and recovery rate. Do your best to get eight hours of sleep a night. Sleep more when you can, so if you're on holiday or have a clear weekend, treat yourself to a few naps — it will benefit you not only by making you train more efficiently, but also by helping you to be more productive in other aspects of your life. If you tell me you don't need more than five hours of sleep a night and don't eat enough calories and no carbs, I don't expect your training to be very successful.

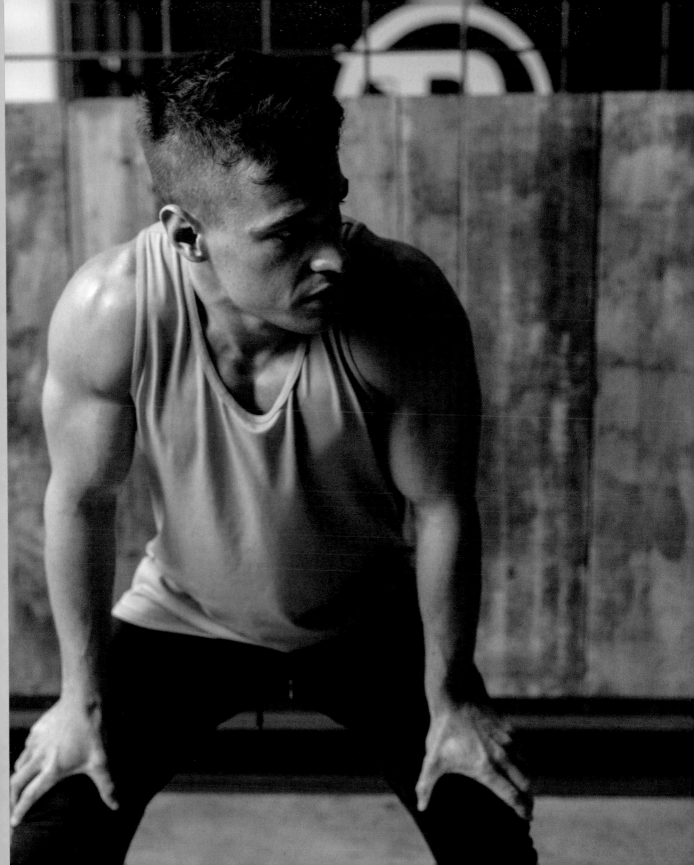

6. AUTO-REGULATING

Another fancy phrase for a very easy concept! This just means that you train based on how you feel on the day or even while in the middle of your session. Training doesn't have to be black and white. It's not a big deal if you don't hit every rep or set to the number (the same principle applies to nutrition; see page 61). So if you're at the gym, you pick up some weights and they feel heavier than usual (and we all know that feeling all too well), don't push it. At the other end of the spectrum, if you're bursting with energy and wellbeing and the weights feel light, add a bit more weight on! So many people push themselves too hard when they're having a bad day because they have too much ego. Pushing through like this can negatively affect your recovery and progress, so listen to your body and ease off, but still do your session to the best of your ability.

7. REST, DON'T RUSH

Whatever level you're at, you know by now that to build lean muscle you need to lift more weight. But don't rush things – allow yourself to recover properly before you hit your next set. Proper rest between sets is what will enable you to lift those extra kilos. This is within reason, though. Twenty minutes is too long to rest – you'd have to set up camp in the gym!

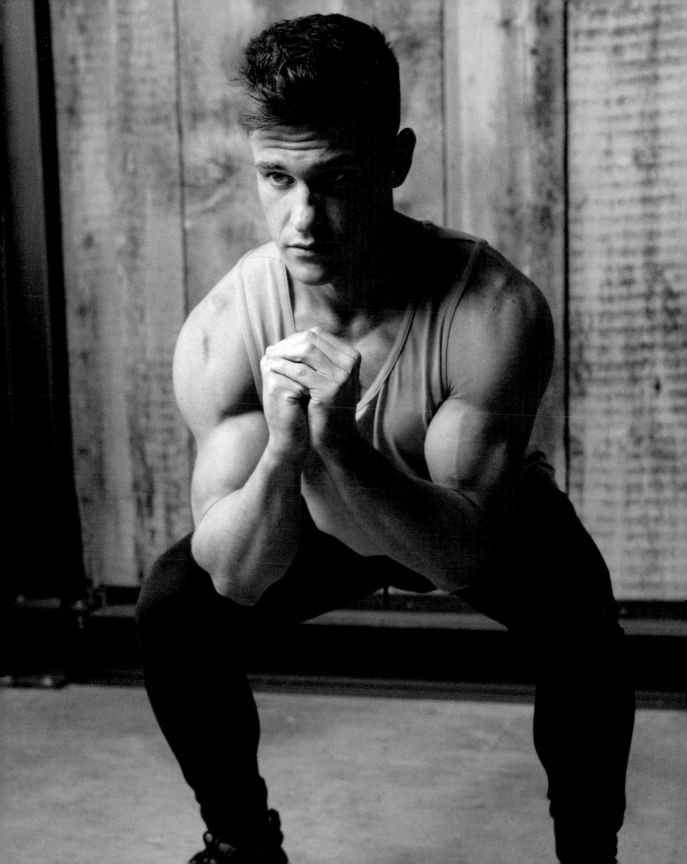

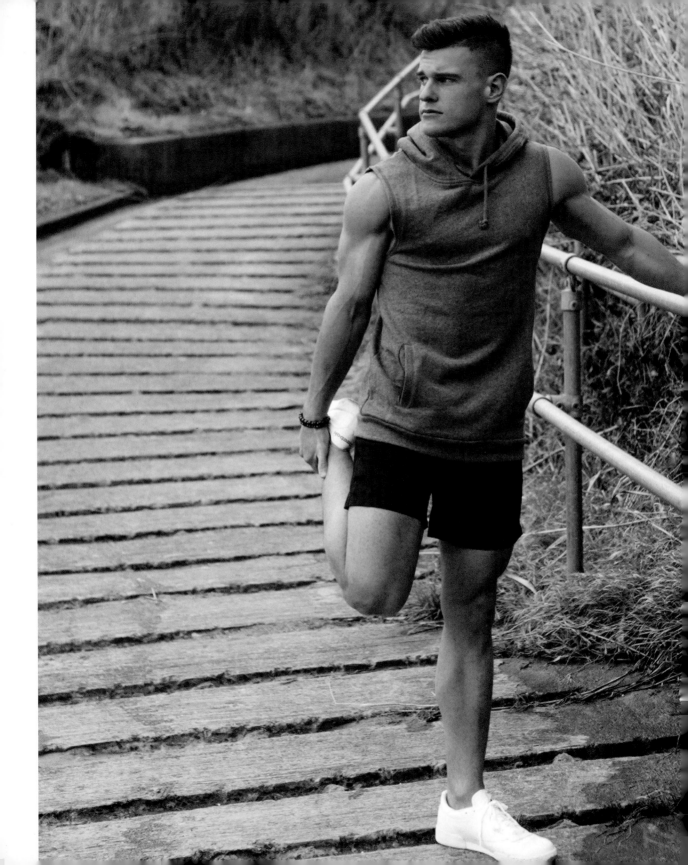

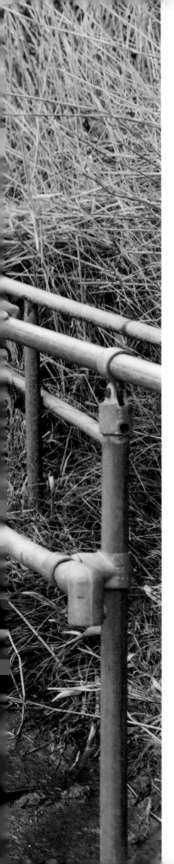

The cardio bit

Let me start this bit by saying that cardio is not exactly necessary for fat loss. When it comes to losing body fat while keeping the most amount of muscle possible, the goal should be to do the least amount of cardio necessary and eat the most calories you can while still getting the job done. As I said in the Nutrition chapter, fat loss is all about creating an energy deficit (see page 39). I strongly recommend combining diet and exercise to create this deficit.

Let's use an example to clarify this. Say somebody needs 2,500 calories a day (maintenance). They want to lose a decent bit of body fat, so they aim to drop it to 2,000 calories a day. They could do one of the following:

> 1. **They could eat 500 calories less per day.**
> 2. **They could eat 250 calories less per day and burn 250 calories more per day.**

I often go for the second option.

For the most part, some cardio every week is good for you – it gets your heart rate up, gets your blood flowing and can burn calories. Let's look into the two main types of cardio that are out there.

HIIT & LISS

I'm sure you've heard the term 'HIIT' being thrown around the fitness circuit, and like most things in this world, when you spell it out it's very simple. HIIT stands for *high-intensity interval training* and involves short, intense bursts of effort followed by a resting period.

An example of a HIIT move could be sprinting:

- You sprint hard (on a treadmill or outside), giving it your all for 30 seconds.
- You rest, walking and breathing slowly for 1 minute.
- Repeat several times.

> "I strongly recommend combining diet and exercise to create this deficit."

On the other hand, LISS stand for *low-intensity steady state* cardio. With LISS, you aim for a lower level of exertion for a longer period.

Examples could include:

- Walking at a moderate pace on an incline treadmill for 30–60 minutes.
- Swimming for 30 minutes.
- Hiking for 30 minutes.

Here's my take on what both have (or don't have) going for them.

HIIT PROS

- As a typical HIIT session will last for only 15–20 minutes, you can get a lot of work done in a small amount of time. As such, it's good for those with time limits.

- It burns calories, continuing even when the session is over.

- Some research suggests that HIIT may be better for fat loss (of course, this needs to be in context).

LISS PROS

- LISS may actually help with recovery. It can be classed as active recovery from more intense exercise and relaxing.

- It's low impact, so it's easier on the joints.

- It doesn't put the nervous system under any stress.

- Anyone can do it — it doesn't require a high fitness or skill level.

- In certain cases you can use your time doing LISS to do something else too, such as listening to podcasts, having phone meetings, etc.

- If you weight train anyway, you're already getting some of the benefits of HIIT (resting and then going again at near full effort), so LISS is a good way to complement that.

HIIT PROS

- This type of intense exercise can be taxing on your recovery and contribute to overtraining.

- It's not suitable for everyone. Those with nagging injuries or those who are overweight may not be able to tackle HIIT.

LISS PROS

- Because it can be time-consuming, it's not good for those with limited time to train.

- Some people may find LISS boring, as it doesn't create the same feel-good hormones that intense exercise does.

WARM UP:

Below is a warm-up routine geared towards a bodyweight HIIT routine. The warm-up applies to both of the routines given and you can also pick some exercises from here for your pre-weight training warm-ups (see page 116).

- Jog on the spot
- Heel kicks
- Bodyweight squats
- Side twists
- Toe touches
- Groin stretches
- Shoulder press-ups
- Loosen up shoulders

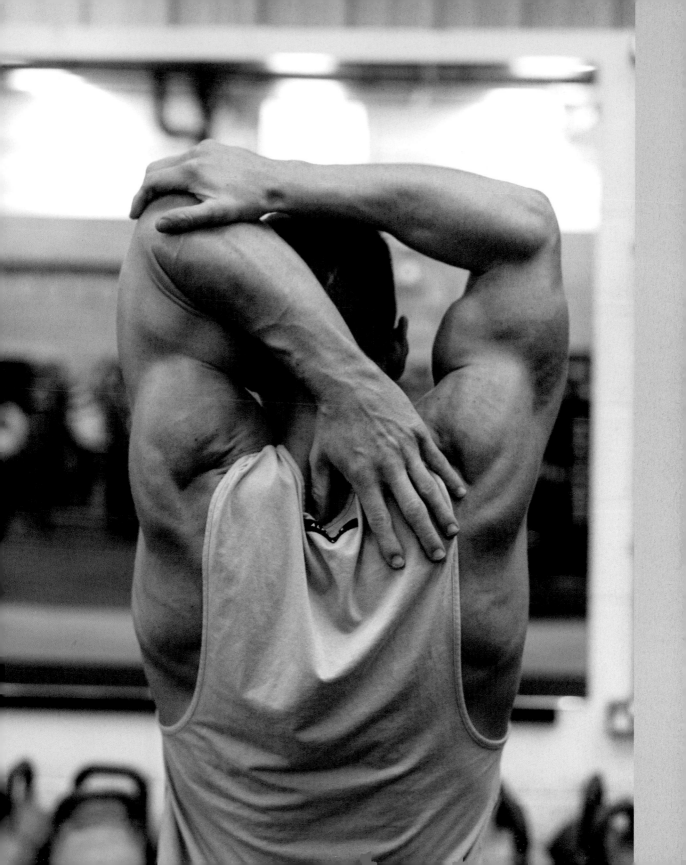

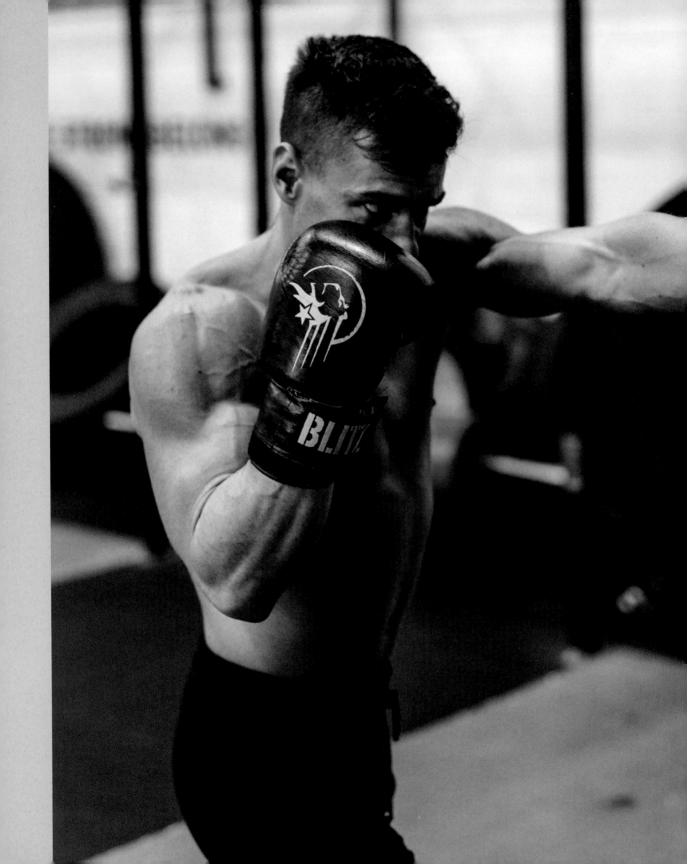

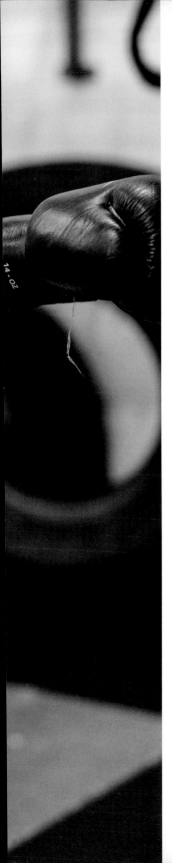

Exercise	Time
Run on the spot	40 seconds (rest 20 seconds)
Burpees	40 seconds (rest 20 seconds)
Bicycle crunches	40 seconds (rest 20 seconds)
Push-ups (add twist for more difficulty)	40 seconds (rest 20 seconds)
Squats (do jump squats for more difficulty)	40 seconds (rest 20 seconds)
Mountain climbers	40 seconds (rest 20 seconds)
Jumping jacks	40 seconds (rest 20 seconds)
Shadow boxing	40 seconds (rest 20 seconds)
Plank	40 seconds (rest 20 seconds)
Close-grip push-ups	40 seconds (rest 20 seconds)
Lunges (add jump for more difficulty)	40 seconds (rest 20 seconds)
Leg raises (abdominals)	40 seconds (rest 20 seconds)
High knees	40 seconds (rest 20 seconds)
Spiderman crunches	40 seconds (rest 20 seconds)
Beach sprints to finish	40 seconds (rest 20 seconds)

Exercise	Reps
Squats	30
Alternating lunges	15 x each leg
Plank	One-minute hold
Push-ups	20
Crunches	20
Burpees	20
Sand sprint	50 metres

TAKE-HOME POINTS

> Pick or create a training regime that you can sustain. The whole thing is pointless if you can't stick to it.

> Be realistic about what you can do per week. There's no point to all this if your workout routine is making you stressed, as you'll only end up putting on more weight!

> Enjoy your training! Remember the age-old tenets: it's more about the journey than the destination; progress is not a straight line.

> Training can be more enjoyable if you do it with other people, so try to find a training buddy. You can keep each other motivated. Getting to know people in your gym can provide a feel-good setting.

> Spread your training properly over the week and work different muscles.

> Don't starve yourself and think it will make you lose weight while training. Eat enough calories to properly sustain your training regime.

> Don't overtrain, as you'll only end up hindering your progress. Balance and listening to your body are key.

> Don't do the same exercises, weights and reps for weeks on end and expect it to make a difference. You need to have a steady progression in your work to see those results.

> Rest enough between sets or you will just wear yourself out and lose progress in the long run.

> Get enough sleep — eight hours a night is ideal.

> Keep hydrated during your workout. Dehydration makes you hungrier, so always have a bottle of water and keep it beside you.

> If you're in doubt about any exercise, ask a trainer for advice.

> Train based on how you feel and learn to listen to your body. This can help you reach your long-term goals and enjoy training more.

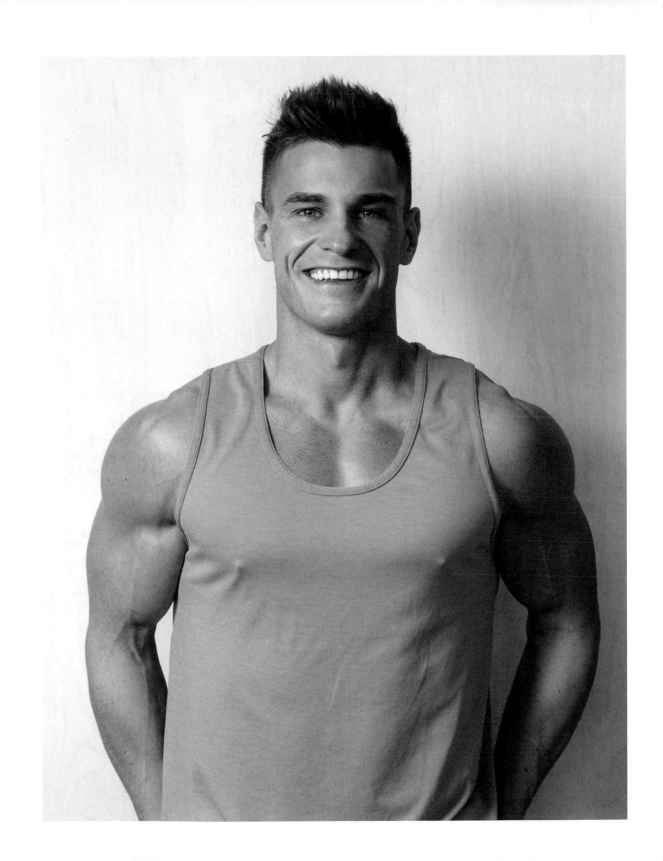

Here are some of my favourite songs to get you amped up for the gym and force out that extra rep when you need it. If you want my full playlist, search for **Rob Lipsett** on Spotify.

Lose Yourself (soundtrack version) **Eminem**

We Own It (Fast & Furious) **2 Chainz, Wiz Khalifa**

Mercy **Kanye West, Big Sean, Pusha T, 2 Chainz**

I Could Be the One Nicktim/radio edit **Avicii, Nicky Romero**

Till I Collapse **Eminem, Nate Dogg**

Somewhere I Belong **Linkin Park**

I Still Can't Stop **Flux Pavilion**

Blame **Zeds Dead, Diplo, Elliphant**

New Level **A$AP Ferg, Future**

Night Rays **Ejeca**

Go F Yourself **Two Feet**

El Chapo (featuring Skrillex) **The Game, Skrillex**

One Man Can Change the World **Big Sean, Kanye West, John Legend**

Bounce Back **Big Sean**

Black Beatles **Rae Sremmurd, Gucci Mane**

Falling (Whethan redo) **Opia, Whethan**

Clique **Kanye West, JAY-Z, Big Sean**

Time **Hans Zimmer**

Black Skinhead **Kanye West**

Adieu (radio edit) **Tchami**

Dreams **NERO, ZHU**

Drone Logic **Daniel Avery**

Look Alive (featuring Drake) **BlocBoy JB, Drake**

No Limit **G-Eazy, A$AP Rocky, Cardi B**

Hypnotize (2014 remastered version) **The Notorious B.I.G.**

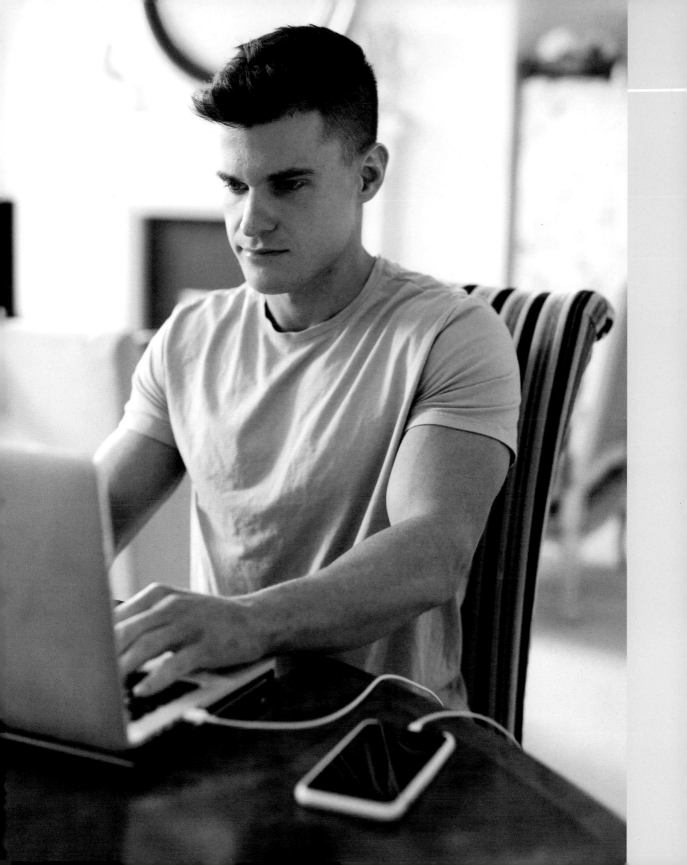

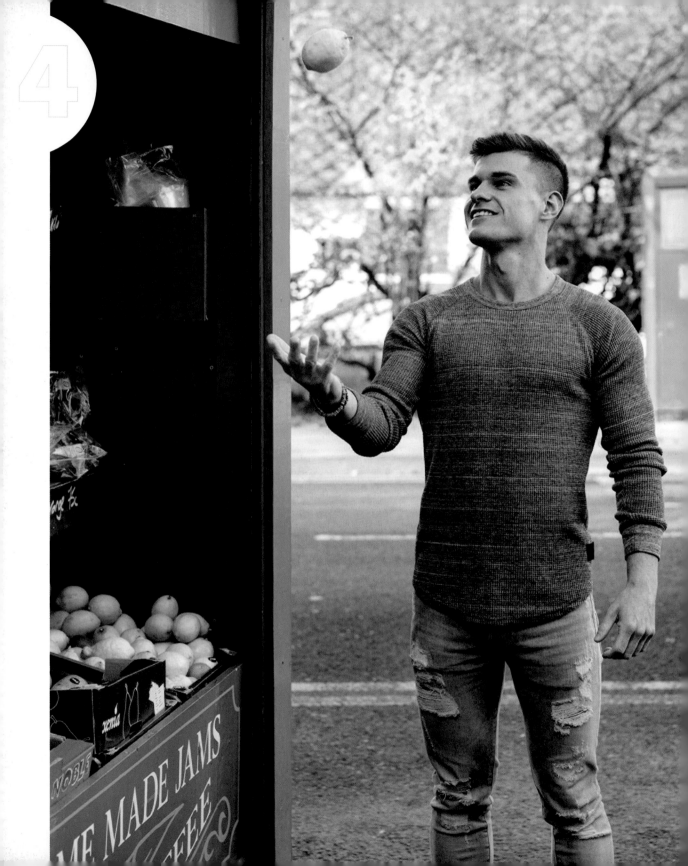

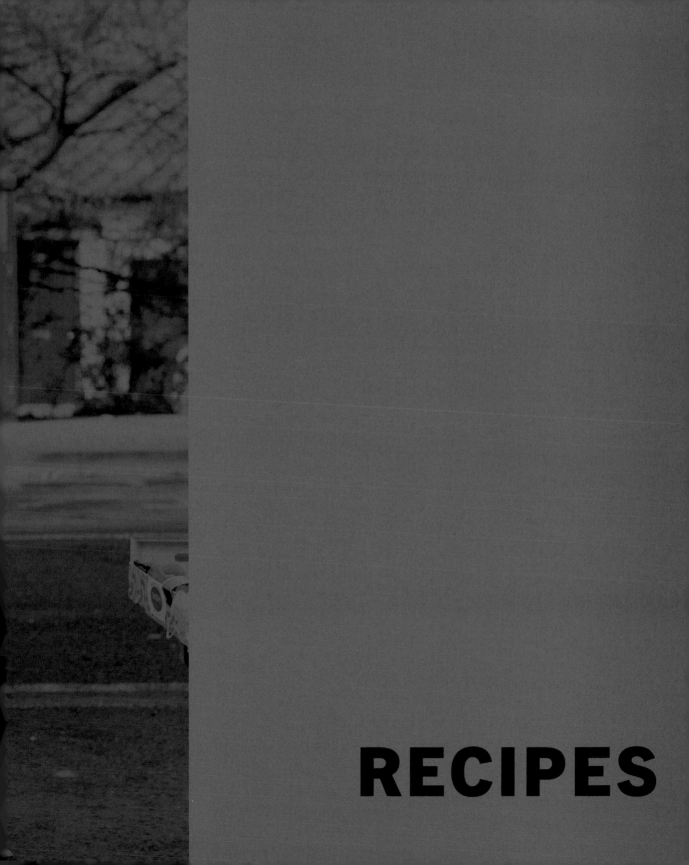

RECIPES

RECIPES

When people ask me for tips on getting ripped, building muscle, getting stronger, improving body composition and making a change to their life, they're always surprised by one of my answers. I say the usual stuff that you know by now: train hard and smart, get your sleep in, hydrate . . . and learn how to cook. It's the cooking part that catches people off guard. 'No, Rob, I don't want to be the next Gordon Ramsay,' they say. 'I just want to get in good shape.'

> "I'm not a nutritionist, dietician or chef, but making a meal that's nutritionally sound and tastes good isn't hard."

Nutrition plays a huge part in getting the body you want, but how do you expect your nutrition to be on point if you can't cook food that's not only nutritious and caters to your goals but tastes good too?

Which brings me to my next point. When I'm asked what the key aspect of any diet is, the first thing I say is sustainability. In this industry I've seen people put on these 'ultra-clean' low-calorie diets that may get them to drop body fat or improve body composition, but can they sustain it? Not a hope. I've seen countless people develop eating disorders from a rigid, overly strict diet (especially those who take part in bodybuilding/physique shows). Once the diet is over, people go back to eating the foods they enjoy (too right!) and undo all their gains.

And that brings us back to cooking. I'm not a nutritionist, dietician or chef, but making a meal that's nutritionally sound and tastes good isn't hard, and both of those are necessary to achieve your goals. These are a few of my go-to recipes that will help you to take your nutrition to the next level and finally start achieving the results you're aiming for.

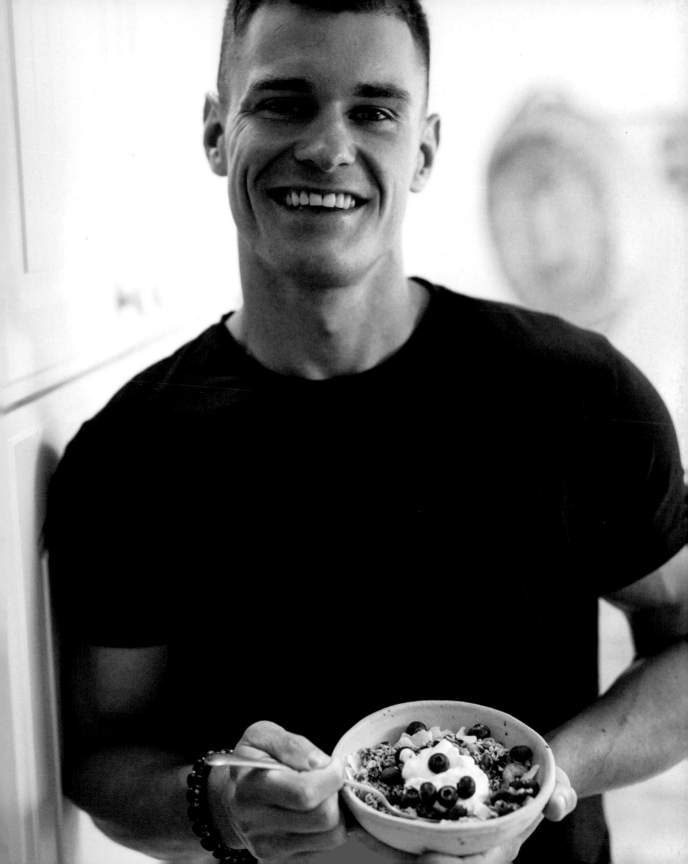

serves

1

Smoothies are perfect for getting you going in the morning or as a snack for post-training recovery. You know the drill by now: for whatever smoothie you want to make, chuck everything into a blender and blitz until smooth. High-powered ones like a NutriBullet work best, but a regular blender will do the job just fine too. Check out my tip on page 202 for freezing bananas to make your smoothies creamy.

smoothies

/Berry & banana smoothie

1 ripe banana
100g frozen strawberries or mixed berries
50g 0% fat high-protein vanilla Greek yoghurt
1 x 30g scoop of protein powder (any flavour)
juice of 2 oranges
splash of milk or water to thin, if needed

/Veggie smoothie

25g baby spinach
2 carrots, peeled and thinly sliced
1 celery stalk, chopped
1 small ripe banana
juice of ½ lime
300ml unsweetened almond milk or water
¼ teaspoon spirulina powder

/PB&J smoothie

1 ripe banana
100g frozen raspberries or strawberries
100g 0% fat high-protein vanilla Greek yoghurt
1 tablespoon smooth peanut butter
200ml high-protein milk

/Blueberry breakfast smoothie

100g frozen blueberries
50g 0% fat high-protein vanilla Greek yoghurt
1 x 30g scoop of protein (any flavour)
20g oats
200ml unsweetened almond milk

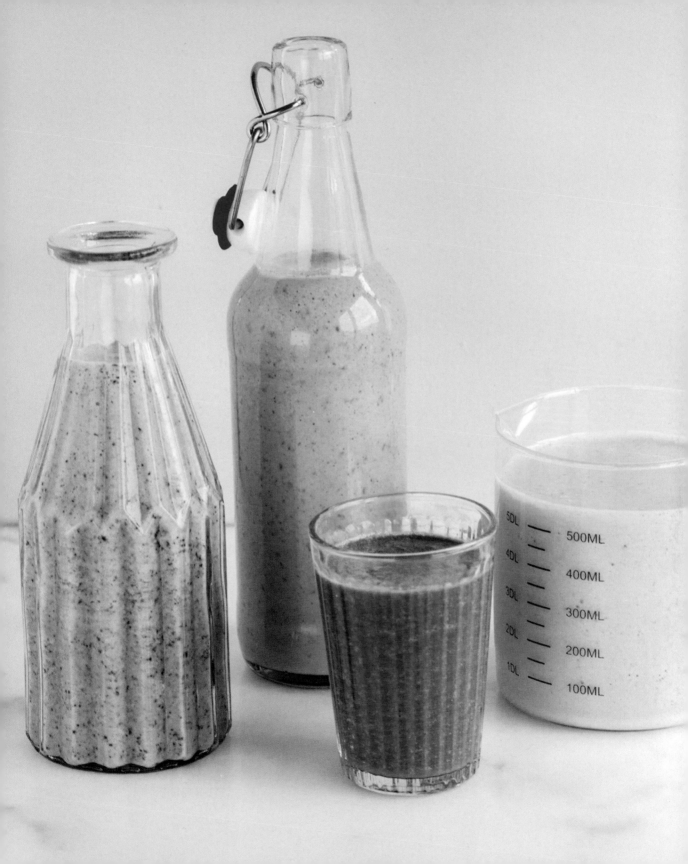

serves

2

This porridge is packed full of good stuff. I make it the night before and put it in the fridge so that all I have to do in the morning is pour it into a pot and heat it up. Soaking the oats overnight also has the added benefit of making them easier to digest. But if planning ahead isn't your strong point, you can make this in the morning and it will be just as good.

fruit & fibre porridge

75g porridge oats
pinch of ground cinnamon
1 ripe banana
1 apple
400ml high-protein milk, plus
    extra to thin if needed
1 x 30g scoop of protein
    powder (any flavour)

To serve (optional):
0% fat high-protein vanilla
    Greek yoghurt
nut butter
chopped almonds
chopped dried fruit, such as
    apricots, dates, raisins or
    cranberries
chopped fresh fruit or berries
honey or maple syrup

Put the oats and a pinch of cinnamon in a medium-sized bowl and mix together.

Using a fork, mash the banana on a chopping board or a plate. Grate the apple, skin and all, on the large holes of a box grater. Add the banana and apple to the oats along with the milk and mix to combine. Cover the bowl with cling film and put in the fridge overnight.

The next morning, pour everything into a pot and cook over a medium heat for about 5 minutes, stirring occasionally, until the porridge is nice and hot. Remove from the heat and stir in the protein powder. The powder will make the porridge thicken up, so add another splash of milk if needed to bring it back to the consistency you like. Divide between two bowls and add your favourite toppings (if using).

breakfast

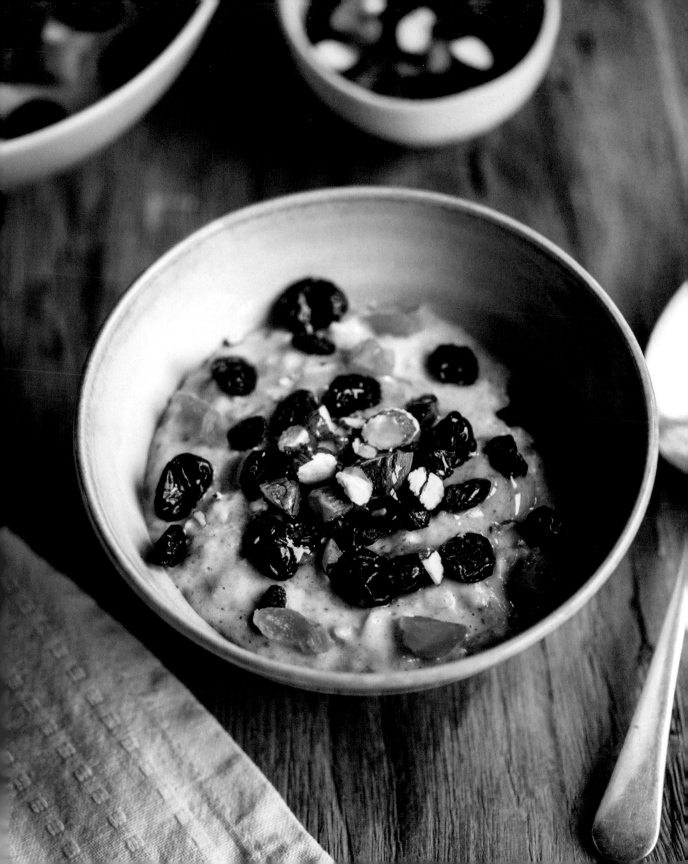

serves
12

Protein isn't always about meat or supplements. Nuts and seeds are good sources of protein too so I load up my granola with them, along with buckwheat groats, which have more protein than other grains and should be available in all health food shops and some of the larger supermarkets. Granola does have a lot of fat, though, so if you want to dial that down, you can leave out the honey and oil altogether, throw everything else straight into a jar, unbaked, and call it muesli instead.

easy-to-make granola

600g jumbo oats
150g buckwheat groats
100g almonds
100g cashews
50g sunflower seeds
50g pumpkin seeds
50g flaxseeds
pinch of salt
200g honey or maple syrup
100g coconut oil
200g dried fruit, such as
　raisins, cranberries, chopped
　apricots or dates
50g coconut flakes

To serve:
0% fat high-protein Greek
　yoghurt
fresh berries or other fruit

Preheat the oven to 150°C.

Put the oats, buckwheat groats, nuts, seeds and a pinch of salt in a large bowl and mix together.

Put the honey or maple syrup and the coconut oil in a small pan set over a medium-low heat. Gently warm together until the coconut oil has melted. Pour this over the dry ingredients and mix until all the oats, nuts and seeds are coated with the oil.

Spread the oat mixture on two baking trays in an even layer. Bake in the oven for 25 minutes, then remove the trays from the oven and give the granola a good stir. Spread it back out in an even layer again, then return the trays to the oven for a further 20 minutes, until the granola is golden brown.

Take the trays out of the oven and stir the granola again so that it doesn't stick to the tray as it cools. Allow to cool completely and crisp up, then stir in the dried fruit and coconut. Serve with yoghurt and some fresh berries or fruit scattered on top.

Stored in a large jar or airtight container, this will keep for up to a month.

breakfast

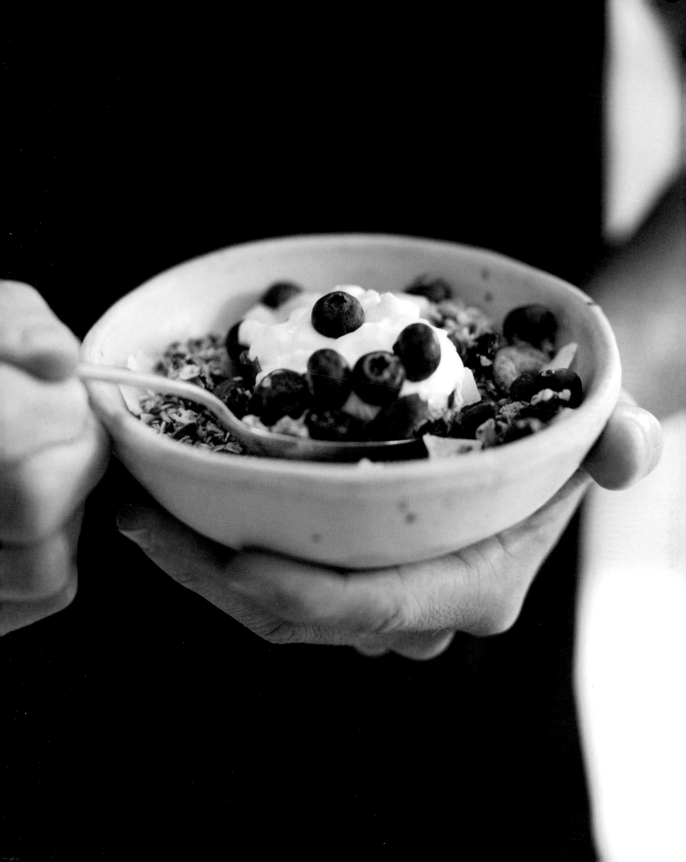

makes
12

These can be served warm, at room temperature or cold, making them a perfect grab-and-go protein hit for any time of the day.

mini frittatas with bacon, spinach & cheddar

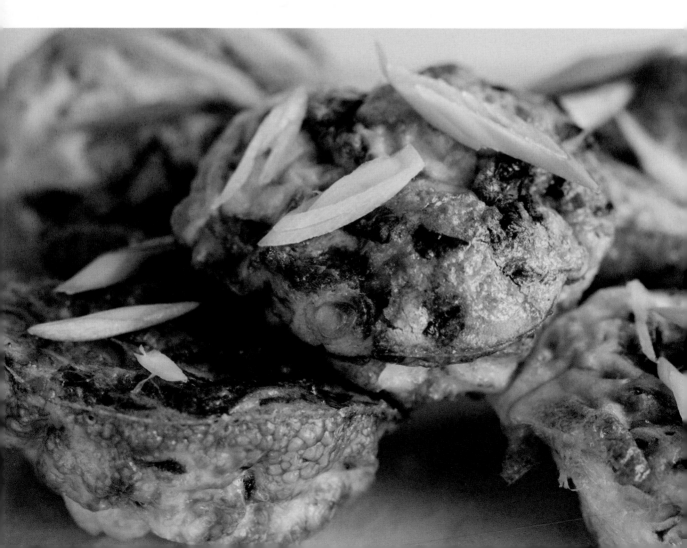

olive oil cooking spray
100g baby spinach
3 slices of bacon
8 eggs
4 egg whites
freshly ground black pepper
2 spring onions, finely chopped,
  plus extra to garnish
50g low-fat Cheddar cheese,
  grated

Preheat the oven to 180°C. Your best option for making sure the frittatas come out of the cases easily is to use a silicone 12-hole muffin tin or lining a regular muffin tin with silicone cases. If you don't have either of those, use paper muffin cases and give each one a spritz of the spray oil. Set the muffin tin on a baking tray to make it easier to put in the oven later on.

Put a large frying pan on a high heat. Add a few spritzes of the olive oil cooking spray, then add the baby spinach and cook for 2 minutes, until it has wilted right down. Remove the pan from the heat and allow the spinach to cool, then transfer to a chopping board and give it a rough chop.

Put a non-stick frying pan over a medium heat. Add a few spritzes of the oil, then add the bacon and cook for 5 minutes, turning it over halfway through, until cooked. Transfer to a chopping board and trim away and discard the fatty rind, then cut the bacon into small pieces.

Put the eggs and egg whites into a medium-sized bowl and season with pepper – you won't need any extra salt because the bacon and cheese are already very salty. Whisk together, then stir in the spinach, bacon, spring onions and cheese.

Transfer the egg mixture to a large jug to make it easier to pour into the muffin tin. Divide the mixture evenly between the 12 holes. Bake in the oven for 20 minutes, until the frittatas have puffed up, the eggs are set and the tops are starting to turn golden brown.

Allow to cool on a wire rack for 5 minutes. Run a knife around the edges of the paper cases to help loosen the frittatas before peeling away the paper, but be prepared for them to stick to the cases, especially on the bottom. They might look a little ragged, but they'll taste great. (If you're using silicone cases, they should come out easily.) Garnish with thinly sliced spring onions if eating right away.

Allow any leftovers to cool completely on the wire rack before storing in an airtight container in the fridge for up to three days.

breakfast

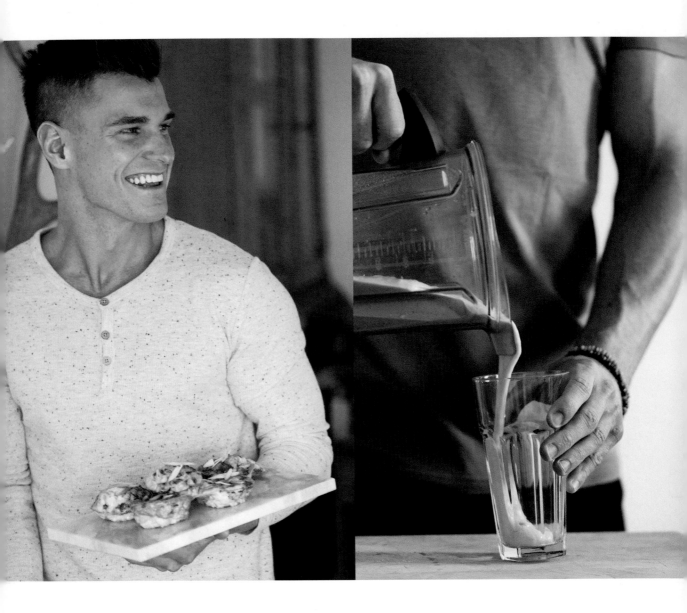

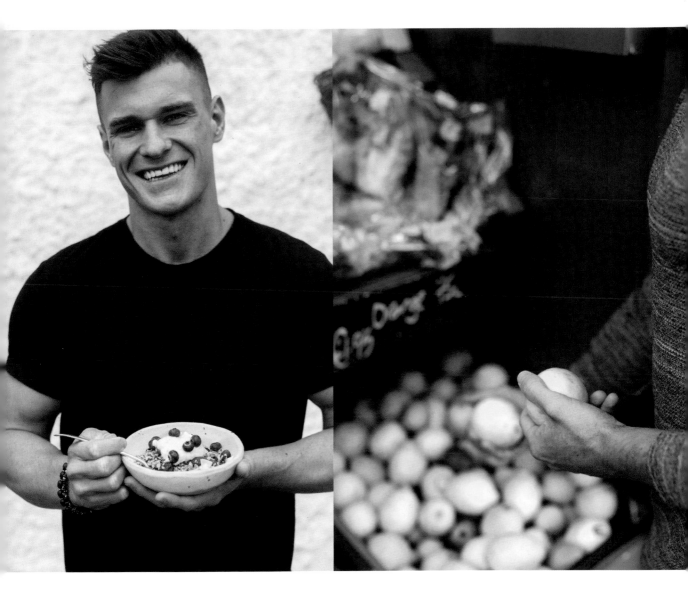

serves

1

My pancake recipe is one of my most popular videos and has racked up nearly 750,000 views on YouTube, so chances are you've seen it or maybe even made them by now. Sometimes you want to change it up for breakfast, though, which is where this stuffed French toast comes in. You need thick slices of bread for this, so buy a whole loaf — ideally wholewheat or wholemeal — and cut it yourself. But if that sounds like too much hassle, use four regular slices of sliced pan and make the French toast like you'd make a sandwich instead of stuffing it. Play around with other fillings, like a high-protein chocolate spread and banana, strawberries and low-fat Quark or cream cheese, or peanut butter and jam for an American-style PB&J twist.

breakfast

stuffed french toast with peanut butter & banana

2 thick slices of bread

2 tablespoons smooth peanut butter

1 large ripe banana, thinly sliced

2 eggs

1 tablespoon milk

½ teaspoon vanilla extract

coconut oil cooking spray

icing sugar, for dusting (optional)

Cut two fat slices from a whole loaf of bread — each slice should be at least 2.5cm thick. Put each slice flat on a cutting board and set your hand on top of it, then use a serrated bread knife to make a horizontal cut through each slice to create a pocket. Cut about three-quarters of the way through, making sure you don't cut all the way through to the other end. You're basically butterflying the bread so that you can open it out like a book. Spread 1 tablespoon of the peanut butter in each pocket, then add a layer of banana slices. Put the eggs, milk and vanilla in a wide, shallow bowl and whisk together until well combined.

Heat a few spritzes of the coconut oil cooking spray in a large non-stick frying pan set over a medium heat. Working with one stuffed slice at a time, put the bread in the bowl and let it soak up the egg mixture for a few seconds before flipping it over and soaking the other side. Make sure the entire slice is coated with the egg mixture and that there aren't any dry patches, then transfer to the hot pan. Cook for 2 or 3 minutes

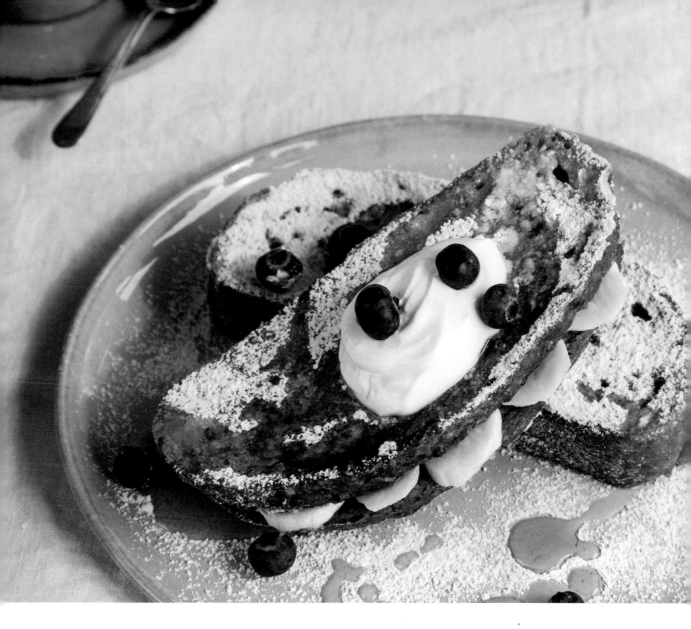

To serve:
2 tablespoons 0% fat
  high-protein vanilla Greek yoghurt,
2 scoops of banana ice cream
  (page 202), to serve (optional)
maple syrup or honey, for
  drizzling
fresh berries, to serve (optional)

without moving the bread, until it's golden brown on the bottom, then flip over and cook the other side for 2 minutes, until that's golden brown too.

Transfer to a plate and dust with icing sugar (if using). Add 1 tablespoon of yoghurt or a scoop of banana ice cream on top of each slice (if using), then drizzle with maple syrup or honey and scatter over some fresh berries.

serves
6

When I was in San Diego one time I ended up crossing over the Mexican border for a wild night in Tijuana. I'd like to say that this was where I discovered this recipe, but truth be told I just like Mexican food in general! Soups are great if you need something hearty on a cold day or if you're feeling a bit under the weather but still need something nutrient-dense and high in protein.

mexican chicken soup

olive oil cooking spray
1 onion, peeled and chopped
2 carrots, peeled and chopped
1 celery stick, chopped
salt and freshly ground black
   pepper
2 garlic cloves, peeled and
   chopped
1 fresh red chilli, deseeded and
   finely chopped (optional)
½ teaspoon ground cumin
   (optional)
½ teaspoon ground coriander
   (optional)
2 chicken fillets, cut into
   bite-sized pieces
750ml chicken stock
1 x 400g tin of black or kidney
   beans, drained and rinsed
1 x 200g tin of salt-free
   sweetcorn, drained and rinsed
juice of 1 lime, plus extra
   wedges to serve

Heat a few spritzes of the olive oil cooking spray in a large saucepan set over a medium heat. Add the onion, carrots, celery and a pinch of salt. Cover the pot with a lid and cook for about 5 minutes, stirring occasionally, until the veg are soft. Add the garlic and chilli along with the cumin and coriander (if using) and cook, uncovered, for 1 minute more.

Add the chicken and cook for 5 minutes, stirring now and then, to give it some colour.

Pour in the stock and bring to the boil, then reduce the heat and simmer for 10 minutes, until the chicken is cooked through. Add the beans and corn and cook for a few minutes to heat them through. Stir in the lime juice, then season to taste with salt and pepper.

Ladle the soup into bowls and garnish with the spring onions, avocado, chilli and coriander. Serve the lime wedges on the side for squeezing over if you want to add a little more zing.

tip

GARNISH WITH: 3 spring onions, thinly sliced; 1 ripe avocado, peeled, stoned and diced; 1 fresh red chilli, deseeded and thinly sliced; ½ bunch of fresh coriander, chopped; 1 lime, cut into wedges

lunch

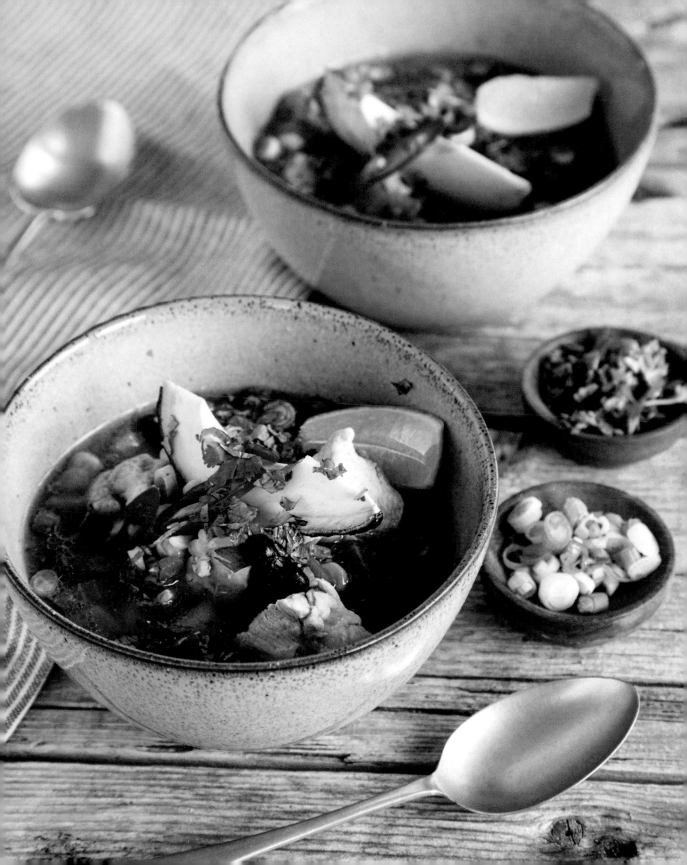

serves
4

This soup is a great way to get in your five a day. It's also good for those times when the cupboards and fridge are bare, with only a few veg knocking around in the crisper, or when you're hanging on till payday and need a cheap and cheerful meal. We've all been there!

root vegetable soup

knob of butter
1 large potato, peeled and
  chopped
1 small onion, peeled and
  chopped
1 large carrot, peeled and
  chopped
1 small parsnip, peeled and
  chopped
1 celery stalk, chopped
salt and freshly ground black
  pepper
1 litre vegetable or chicken
  stock
splash of milk (optional)
0% fat high-protein Greek
  yoghurt, to garnish
alfalfa sprouts, to garnish

Melt the butter in a large saucepan set over a medium heat. Add all the veg and stir to coat them in the butter. Add a good pinch of salt, then cover the pan with a lid and sweat the veg for 10 minutes, until softened.

Pour in the stock, cover the pan again and cook for 15 minutes more, until all the veg are completely tender. Use a hand-held blender to blitz the soup until it's smooth. If you want to thin it a bit, add a splash of milk and blend again until it's the consistency you want. Season to taste with salt and pepper.

To serve, ladle into warmed bowls and garnish with a dollop of yoghurt and a small pinch of alfalfa sprouts.

lunch

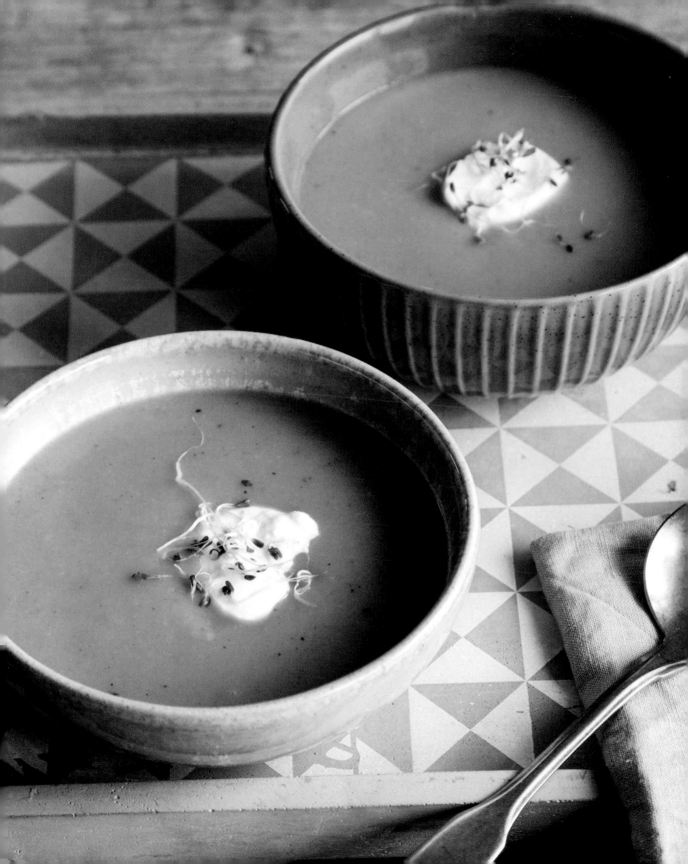

serves
4-6

Portion this up into airtight containers and stash them in the fridge, ready to have on hand for a few days' worth of lunches. A word of warning though: be sure to let the cooked chicken, pasta and peas cool down completely before adding them to the yoghurt pesto sauce, otherwise any residual heat can make the yoghurt turn a bit clumpy.

creamy chicken, pea & pesto pasta salad

lunch

2 large chicken fillets
salt and freshly ground black
  pepper
500g wholewheat fusilli or
  penne pasta
250g frozen peas
300g low-fat Greek yoghurt
3–4 tablespoons shop-bought
  pesto
100g pine nuts
fresh basil leaves, to garnish
  (optional)

To poach the chicken, put the fillets in a medium-sized saucepan and cover with plenty of cold water, then season the water with a generous pinch of salt and pepper. Set the pan over a high heat and bring to the boil, then reduce the heat, cover the pan and simmer for about 15 minutes, until the chicken is completely cooked through. Transfer the chicken to a plate and allow to cool completely, then cut into small bite-sized pieces.

Meanwhile, bring a large pot of salted water to the boil. Add the pasta and cook according to the packet instructions, then drain and allow to cool completely.

Bring a separate medium-sized pan of salted water to the boil. Add the peas and cook for 3 minutes, then drain and run them under the cold tap to lock in their bright green colour. Allow to cool completely.

Put the yoghurt and pesto in a large mixing bowl and stir to combine. Add the cooled chicken, pasta and peas along with the pine nuts and stir until everything is coated with the creamy pesto sauce. Add a little more yoghurt or pesto (or both) if you want more sauce. Season to taste with salt and pepper, then garnish with fresh basil leaves (if using).

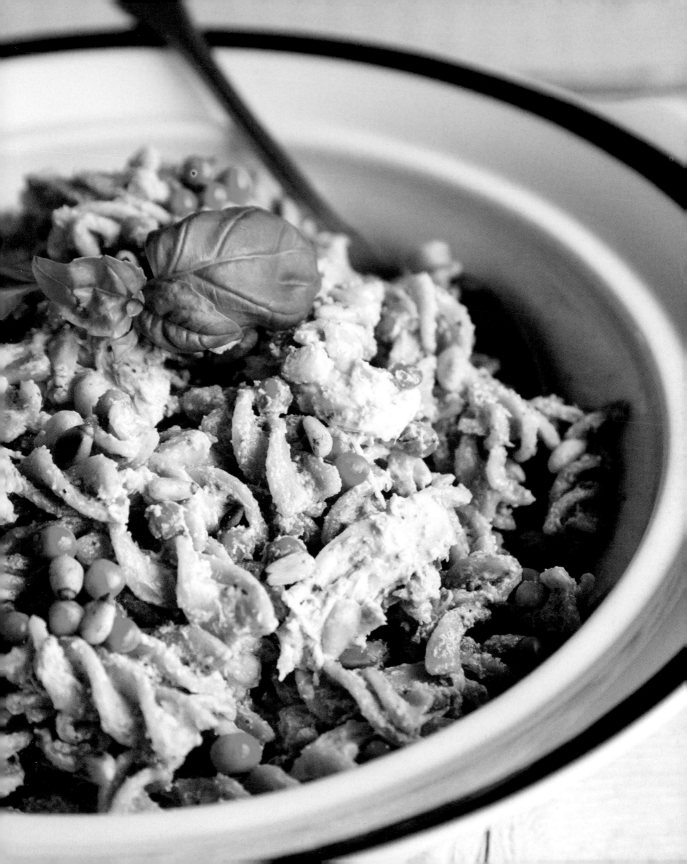

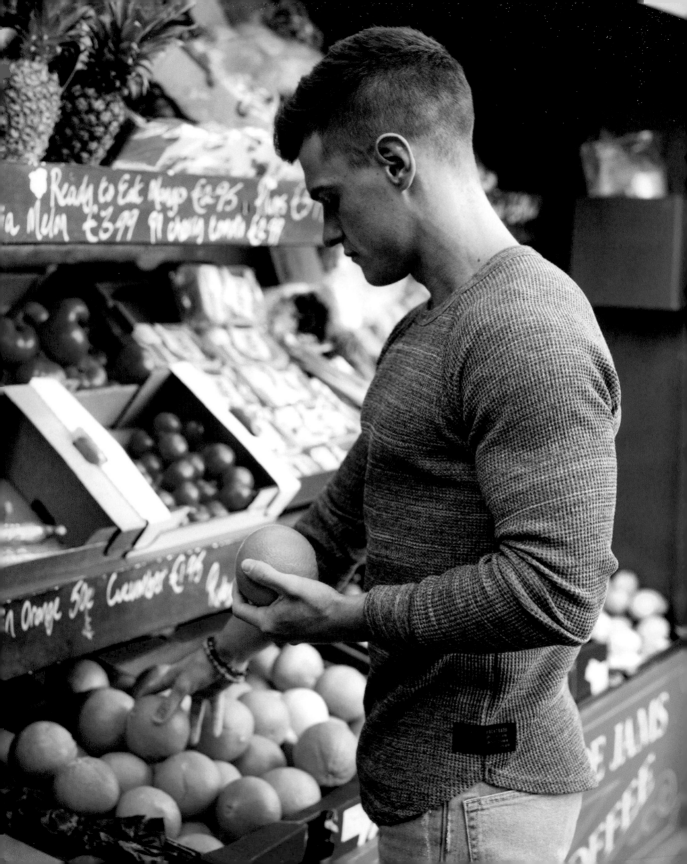

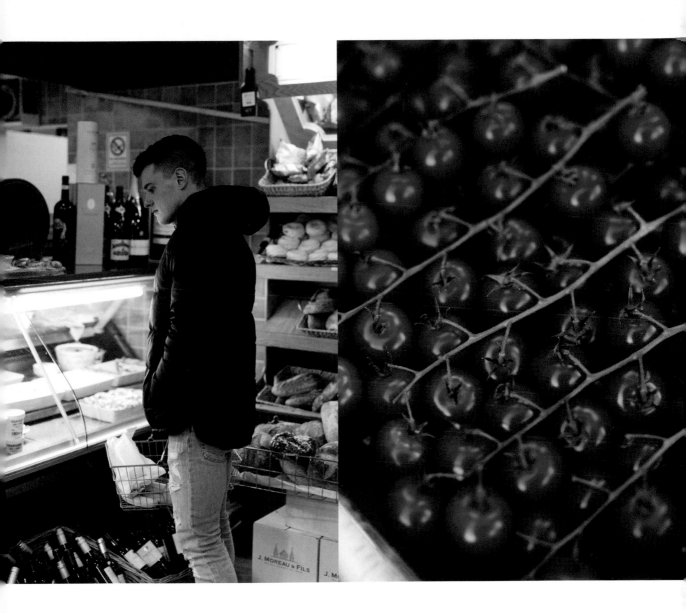

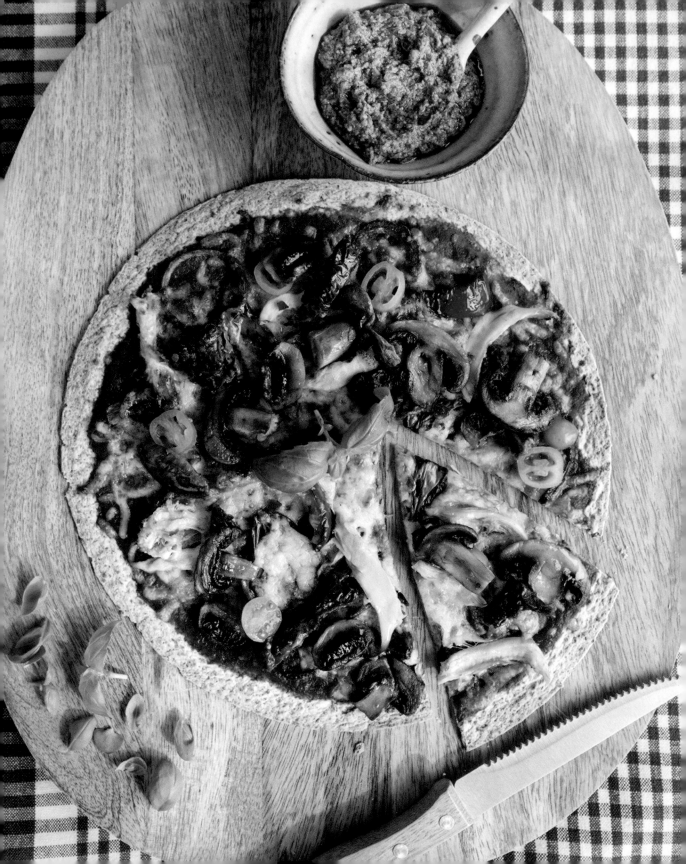

makes

1

The key to any diet is sustainability, so being able to enjoy some of your favourite foods, like pizza, plays a big part in being able to stick with it. This super-quick and easy recipe makes one tortilla pizza, so scale it up to make however many you want. Add whatever other toppings you like, but don't overdo it or the tortilla won't be able to take the weight – less is more! Or go ahead and make this into a regular pizza and adjust the amount of the toppings and the cooking time accordingly. I use the stoneground Pizza da Piero bases, which are Irish-made and available in good delis or some supermarkets. If you want to get in even more protein, use a high-protein cheese, which you can buy online.

macro-friendly pizza

olive oil cooking spray
1 wholemeal tortilla
2 tablespoons shop-bought pizza
   sauce
50g grated mozzarella, low-fat
   Cheddar cheese or a mix of the two
a few fresh basil leaves (optional)

TOPPING IDEAS:
- roasted red peppers from a jar
- halved Peppadew peppers
- chopped cooked ham
- shredded cooked chicken
- sautéed mushrooms with
   garlic and fresh thyme
- wilted baby spinach
- quartered cherry tomatoes
- chopped sun-dried tomatoes
- thinly sliced red onions
- roasted veg with shop-bought
   basil pesto

lunch

Preheat the oven to 200°C.

Spritz a pizza pan or baking tray with the olive oil cooking spray, then put the tortilla on the pan. Put the pizza sauce in the middle of the tortilla and use the back of a spoon to spread it over the tortilla, making sure you leave a thin edge clear for the crust.

Put the grated cheese in a mound in the middle of the tortilla. Use the palm of your hand to spread it out evenly across the tortilla, again leaving the edges clear for the crust.

Add any other toppings you want at this stage, but keep in mind that just like a regular pizza, you should aim to get a good balance of toppings across the tortilla and you shouldn't overload it.
Put the tortilla in the oven and bake for about 10 minutes, until the tortilla base is crisp and the cheese has melted. If you're adding fresh basil, put it on after the pizza comes out of the oven. Allow to stand for 1 minute, then cut into quarters.

When I was a student trying to cook delicious yet low-cost meals, some of my go-to foods were eggs and potatoes – and they're still a staple part of my diet. This Spanish tortilla is a great way to get in some healthy sources of fat, filling carbohydrates and of course a complete protein source too.

spanish tortilla

300g baby potatoes (about 6 small potatoes)

4 teaspoons olive oil

1 large onion, peeled and thinly sliced

salt and freshly ground black pepper

2 garlic cloves, peeled and chopped

8 eggs

1 tablespoon finely chopped fresh flat-leaf parsley

green salad, to serve

Put the potatoes in a medium-sized saucepan and cover with cold water. Bring to the boil, then reduce the heat and simmer for 7 to 10 minutes, depending on how big the potatoes are, until the spuds are just tender when you test them with the tip of a sharp knife. Don't overcook them or they won't keep their shape when sliced. Drain and allow to cool. When they're cool enough to handle, slice thinly and set aside.

Preheat the oven to 180°C.

Heat 1 teaspoon of the olive oil in a large ovenproof, non-stick frying pan set over a medium heat. Add the onion and a good pinch of salt and cook for about 10 minutes, stirring occasionally, until softened. Add the garlic and cook for 1 minute more, then remove from the heat.

Whisk the eggs in a large bowl with a pinch of salt and pepper. Add the sliced potatoes, onion mixture and parsley and give everything a good stir. Wipe out the frying pan and add the remaining 3 teaspoons of olive oil. Put the pan over a medium heat to let the oil warm up, then pour in the egg mixture, making sure the potatoes and onions are evenly distributed throughout the pan.

Transfer the pan to the oven and cook for about 30 minutes, until the tortilla has puffed up and is set in the centre. Remove from the oven and allow to cool a little before loosening the edges and base away from the pan with a spatula. Slide it out of the pan on to a large serving platter or cutting board and scatter with parsley. Cut into wedges and serve warm or at room temperature with a green salad on the side.

lunch

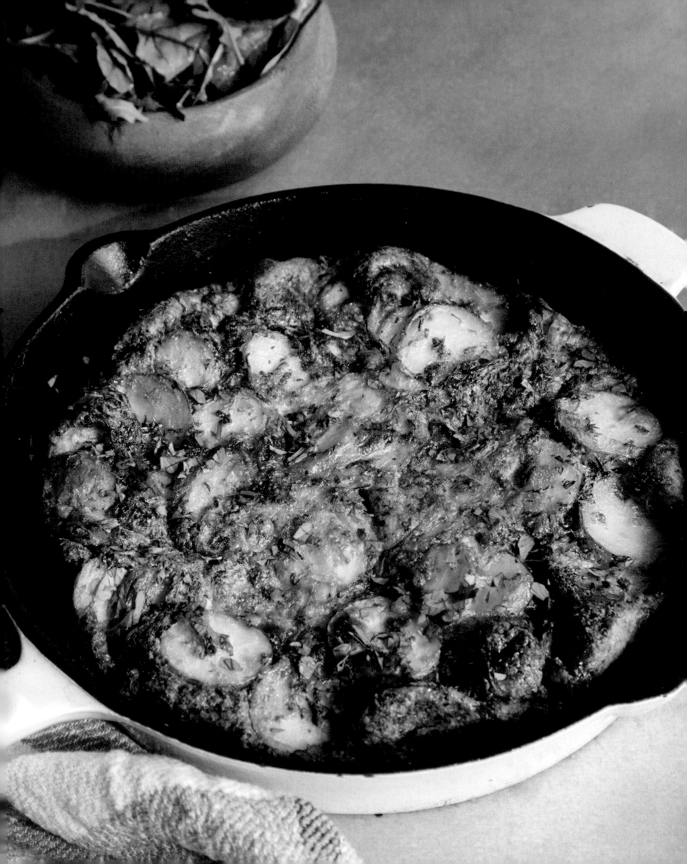

serves
4-6

People often ask me what I eat the most, and this is it. In my opinion, it's the perfect meal and a great way to get in lots of quality macros. And the best thing about a burrito bowl is that you can customize it however you want. Don't have fresh cherry tomatoes? Use a good shop-bought salsa instead. Want to pack in even more protein? Use quinoa instead of rice. Trying to keep your carbs down? Leave the rice out altogether. Don't have all the spices? Grab a jar of fajita seasoning from the shop. You get the idea.

burrito bowl

250g basmati rice
olive oil cooking spray
1 onion, peeled and finely diced
1 red pepper, finely diced
2 garlic cloves, peeled and
  finely chopped
400g lean beef or turkey mince
½ teaspoon ground cumin
½ teaspoon ground coriander
¼ teaspoon smoked paprika
¼ teaspoon chilli powder
salt and freshly ground black
  pepper
1 tablespoon chopped fresh
  coriander, to garnish

Cook the rice according to the packet instructions. Keep it warm if you'll be eating this right away or let it cool completely if you'll be packing it into a lunchbox.

Heat a few spritzes of the olive oil cooking spray in a large non-stick frying pan set over a medium heat. Add the onion and red pepper and cook for about 5 minutes, until softened. Add the garlic and cook for just 1 minute, then add the beef or turkey mince, spices and a good pinch of salt and pepper and cook for 8 to 10 minutes, stirring occasionally, until the mince is browned and cooked through. Taste and add more salt and pepper if you think it needs it.

Now it's time to build your burrito bowl into something Instagram-worthy! Add separate mounds of the rice and beef to a large shallow bowl, like a pasta bowl, then add whatever other optional extras you're using in separate piles until the bowl is full. Top with some grated Cheddar or high-protein cheese, one or two spoonfuls of Greek yoghurt or Quark, as much hot sauce as you can handle and lime wedges on the side for squeezing over, then sprinkle everything with the chopped fresh coriander.

If you want this to last for a few days' worth of lunches, let the rice and beef cool and get a little assembly line going to pack all your ingredients into a few airtight containers.

dinner

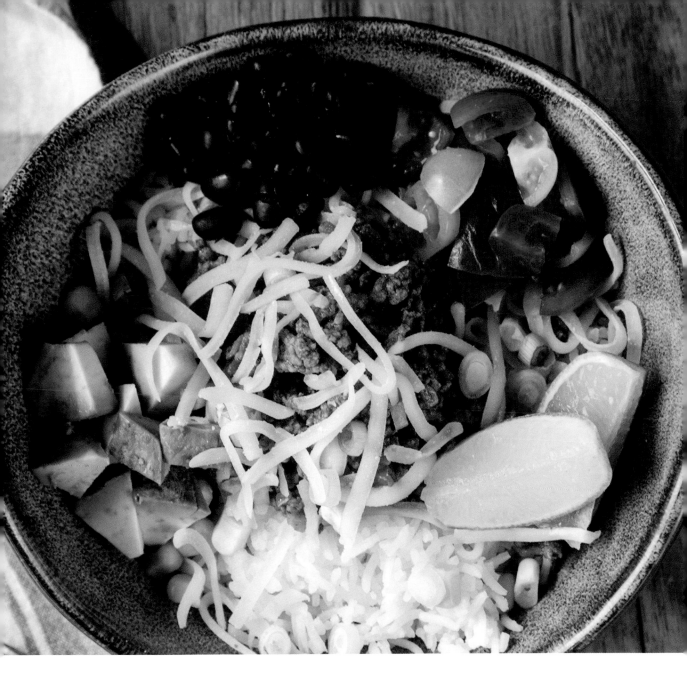

 OPTIONAL EXTRAS: 1 x 400g tin of black or kidney beans, drained and rinsed; 1 x 200 tin of salt-free sweetcorn,drained and rinsed; 12 cherry tomatoes, halved, or shop-bought tomato salsa; 4 spring onions, thinly sliced; 1 ripe avocado, peeled, stoned and sliced; handfuls of baby salad leaves; grated low-fat Cheddar or high-protein cheese; low-fat Greek yoghurt or Quark cheese; sriracha or Tabasco sauce; lime wedges

serves
4

I was on holiday in Thailand recently and loved the fresh flavours of the food there. Even if it's cold and raining in Dublin, this dinner takes me back to the beaches of Kho Tao. I like to keep this carb free by serving the pork in lettuce cups, but you could have it on top of some boiled basmati rice or thin rice noodles if you need something more substantial.

thai pork lettuce cups

coconut oil cooking spray
450g pork mince
2 tablespoons lime juice
1 tablespoon fish sauce
pinch of caster sugar
4 tablespoons finely chopped
  fresh mint, basil or coriander
  (or better yet, a mix of all
  three)
2–3 heads of baby gem
  lettuce, broken into
  individual leaves
4 cherry tomatoes, finely
  diced
2 spring onions, thinly sliced
½ cucumber, seeds scooped
  out and finely diced
½ fresh red chilli, deseeded
  and thinly sliced (optional)

Heat a few spritzes of the coconut oil cooking spray in a large non-stick frying pan set over a high heat. Add the pork and cook, stirring constantly, for 5 to 7 minutes, until cooked through and all the liquid has evaporated.

Put the lime juice, fish sauce and sugar in a small bowl and whisk together, then add to the pork and cook for 1 or 2 minutes more. Take the pan off the heat and stir in the fresh herbs.

To serve, put a spoonful of the pork in individual baby gem cups. Top each one with small amounts of the cherry tomatoes, spring onions, cucumber and chilli (if using) to make the perfect bite.

dinner

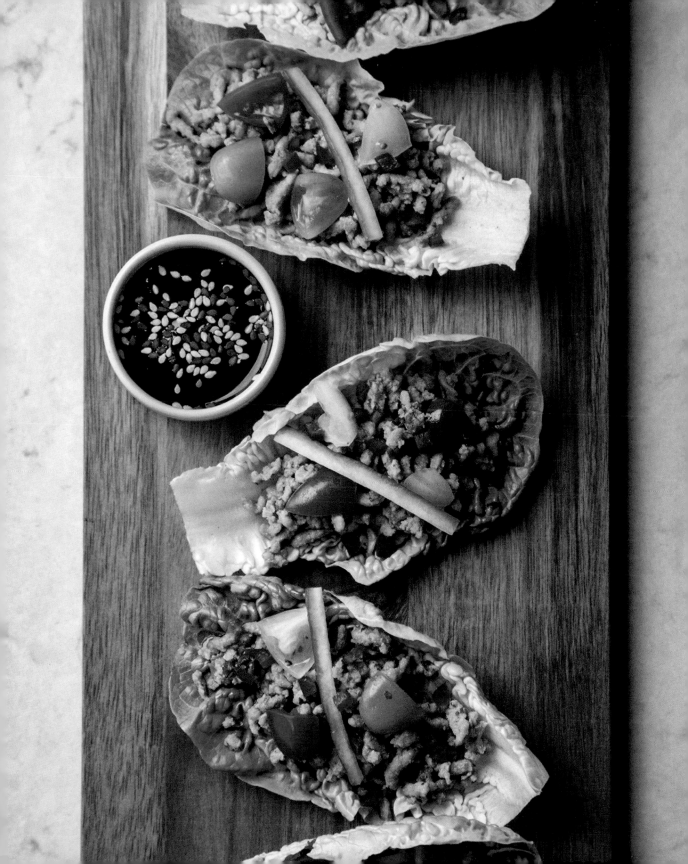

makes

6

Turkey mince is a versatile lean protein, but let's be honest, it can be pretty dry and bland. I give these burgers a boost by mixing in some light mayo.

turkey burgers

1 egg

2 tablespoons light mayonnaise

400g turkey mince

100g fresh breadcrumbs

2 spring onions, white and green parts finely chopped

salt and freshly ground black pepper

olive oil cooking spray

6 pitta breads or burger buns, to serve

shop-bought frozen sweet potato fries, to serve (optional)

If you're serving the burgers with shop-bought frozen sweet potato fries, get them going first – cook according to the packet instructions.

Put the egg and mayo in a medium-sized bowl and whisk together, then add the turkey mince, breadcrumbs, spring onions and a generous pinch of salt and pepper. Use your hands to mix everything together until just combined, but the trick here is to handle the burgers as little as possible so that they don't toughen up. Divide into six equal portions and form into burgers. If you're using pitta bread, make sure the burgers are a small enough size that they'll fit into them.

Heat a few spritzes of the olive oil cooking spray in a large non-stick frying pan set over a medium heat. Add the burgers and cook for 5 minutes on each side, until completely cooked through.

Meanwhile, put the pittas or burger buns on a baking tray and toast in a hot oven for a few minutes. If using pittas, when they're cool enough to handle, cut a slit into the top and open it out to make a pocket that will fit the burgers.

Serve the burgers in the pitta breads or burger buns with any of the optional extras you like and the oven-baked sweet potato fries on the side.

tip

OPTIONAL EXTRAS: light mayonnaise; baby gem or butterhead lettuce leaves; 1 ripe avocado, peeled, stoned and sliced; ½ red onion, peeled and thinly sliced into rings; 2 ripe tomatoes, sliced

dinner

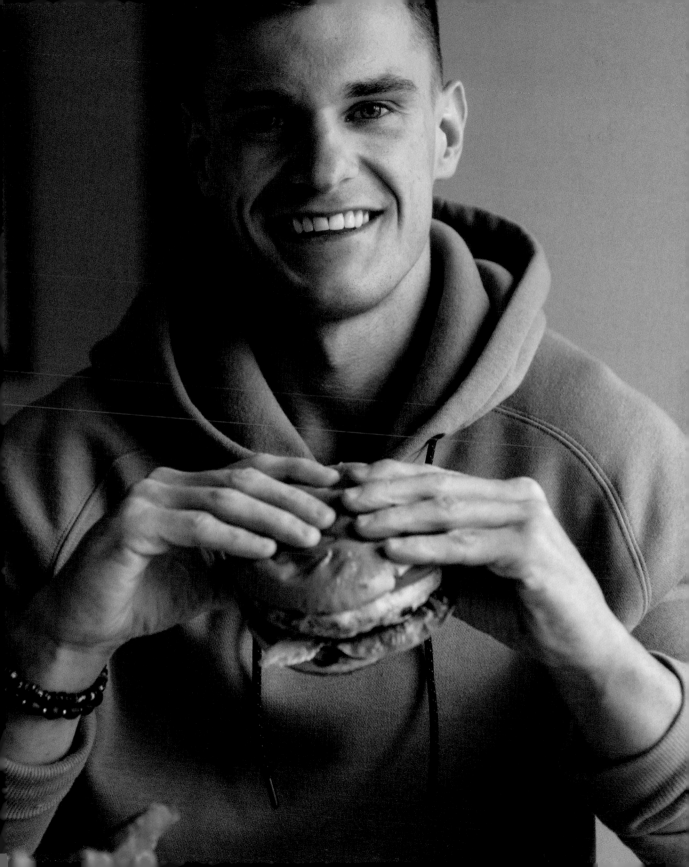

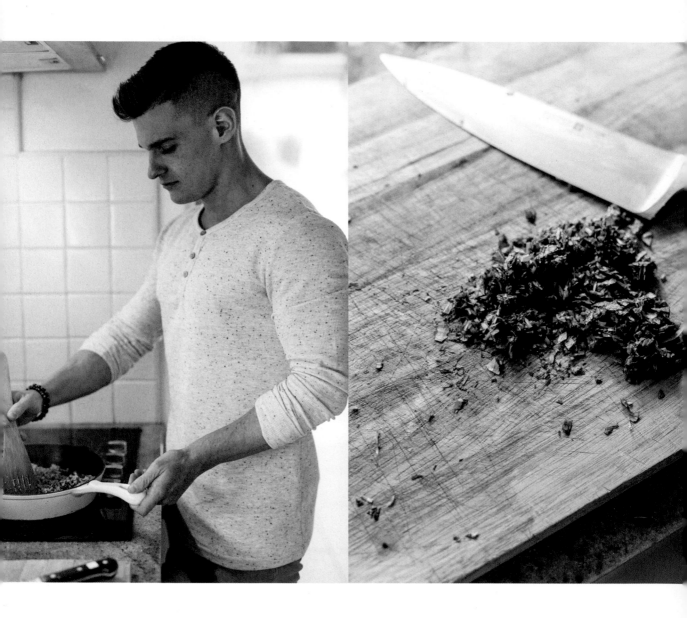

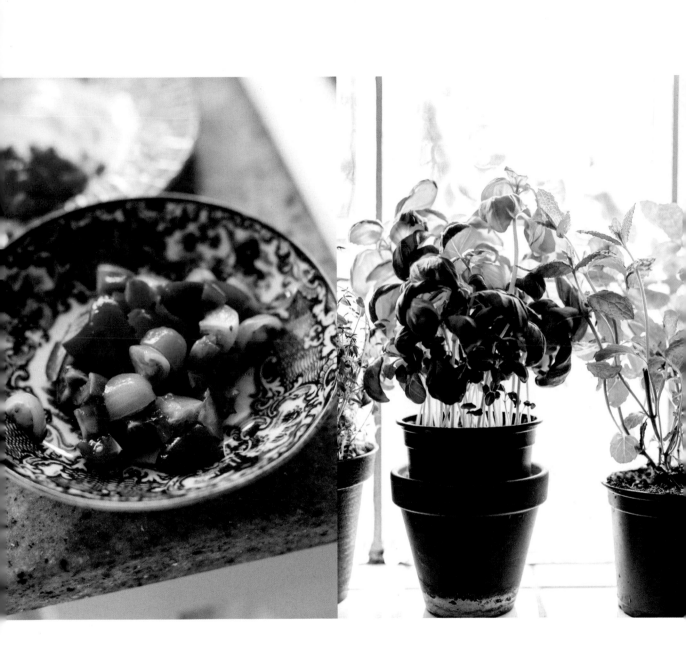

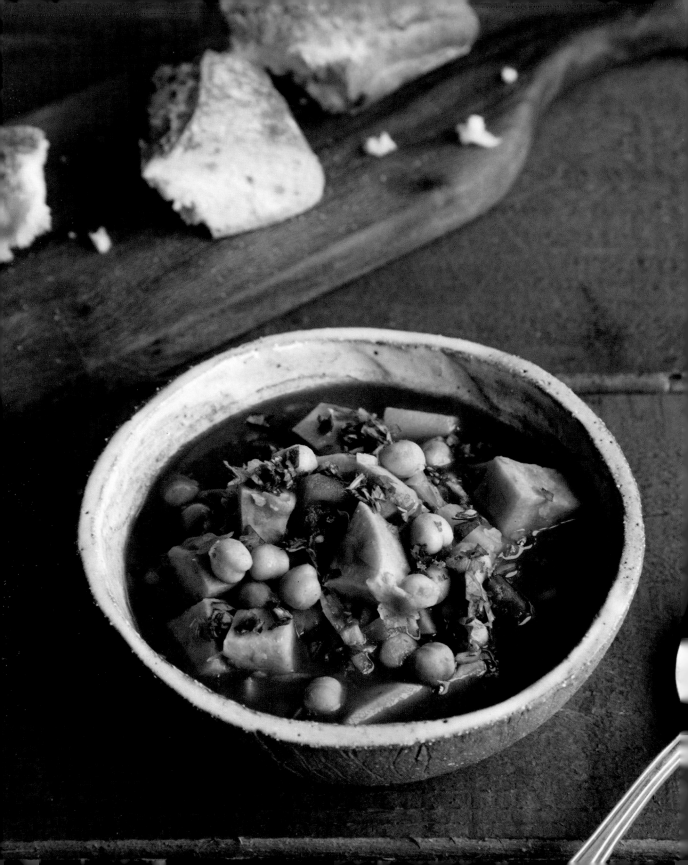

serves

4

This vegetarian stew is a great option for Meatless Monday, but you could bulk it out with some extra protein, such as cooked shredded chicken, cooked chopped ham or pan-fried cubes of chorizo.

smoky sweet potato & chickpea stew

olive oil cooking spray

1 onion, peeled and chopped

3 garlic cloves, peeled and
chopped

2 teaspoons smoked paprika

1 teaspoon harissa or chilli powder

3 sweet potatoes, peeled and
chopped into bite-sized pieces

2 x 400g tins of chickpeas, drained
and rinsed

1 x 400g tin of chopped tomatoes

500ml vegetable or chicken stock

1 tablespoon chopped fresh
coriander or flat-leaf parsley, to
garnish

crusty bread, to serve

Heat a few spritzes of the olive oil cooking spray in a large saucepan set over a medium-low heat. Add the onion, cover the pan and cook for about 10 minutes, until the onion is completely softened. Add the garlic, smoked paprika and harissa or chilli powder and cook, uncovered, for 1 minute more.

Add the sweet potatoes, chickpeas, tomatoes and stock.

Bring to the boil, then reduce the heat and simmer, uncovered, for 20 to 30 minutes, until the sweet potatoes are completely tender.

Serve in bowls garnished with the fresh coriander or parsley and a hunk of crusty bread on the side to mop up all the stew.

dinner

serves

4

Who said cooking has to be hard or time-consuming? If you can chop an onion and open a few tins and jars, you can make this curry and have it on the table in half an hour. No excuses!

quick fish curry

coconut oil cooking spray

1 onion, chopped

3 tablespoons of your favourite curry paste

1 x 400ml tin of low-fat coconut milk

450g hake fillets, skinned, boned and cut into bite-sized chunks

200g frozen prawns

To serve:

1 fresh red chilli, deseeded and thinly sliced

1 tablespoon finely chopped fresh coriander

boiled basmati rice or naan bread

1 lime, cut into wedges

Heat a few spritzes of the coconut oil cooking spray in a large saucepan set over a medium heat. Add the onion, cover the pan and cook, stirring occasionally, for about 10 minutes, until softened. Add the curry paste and cook, uncovered, for a few minutes more.

Shake the tin of coconut milk before you open it to disperse the solids that settle on top, then pour it into the pan. Bring up to a simmer, then add the hake and prawns and cook for 5 minutes, until the hake is cooked through and flakes apart easily when you gently press it with a fork.

Divide between your serving bowls and scatter the chilli and fresh coriander on top. Serve with boiled basmati rice or naan bread to soak up all the sauce, and lime wedges on the side for squeezing over.

dinner

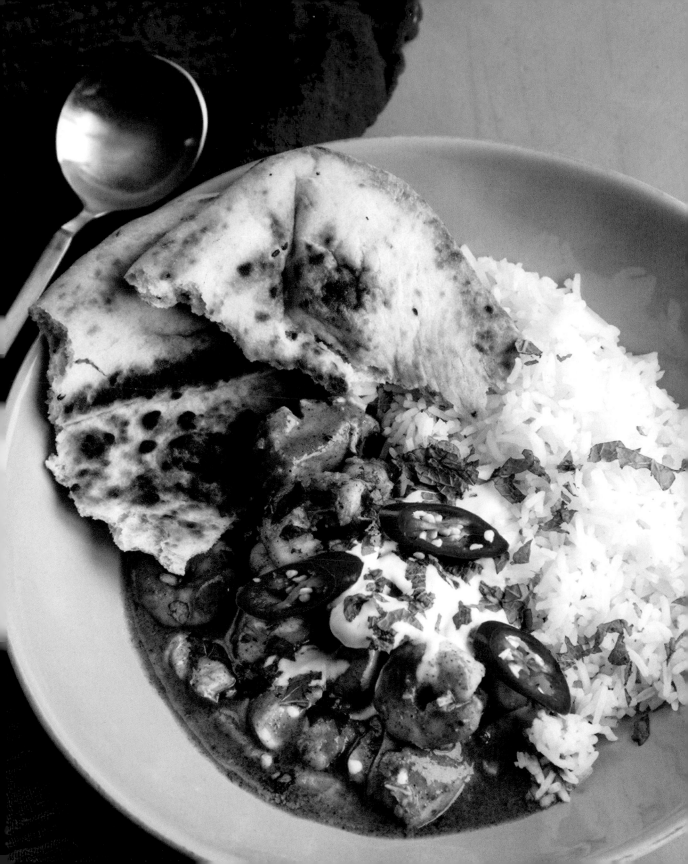

makes
22

You can't beat the combination of chocolate and peanut
butter, but you could use any nut butter in these.

chocolate, chia & peanut butter protein balls

30g oats
1 x 30g scoop of chocolate
   protein powder
3 tablespoons smooth peanut
   butter
2 tablespoons honey
1 tablespoon chia seeds
1 tablespoon almond milk
pinch of salt
sesame seeds, desiccated
   coconut and/or cocoa powder,
   to coat

Put the oats, protein powder, peanut butter, honey, chia seeds, almond
milk and a pinch of salt in a food processor or blender and blitz until
it comes together into a ball. If you think it looks a bit dry, add another
teaspoon of milk and blend again.

First run your hands under the cold tap to dampen them so that the
mixture doesn't stick to your hands too much. Use a teaspoon to scoop
out small portions – don't be tempted to make them any bigger, they're
meant to be small bites – and roll into a smooth ball between the palms
of your dampened hands.

Put the sesame seeds, desiccated coconut and/or cocoa powder in a
bowl. Working with one ball at a time, toss them in the bowl until coated
all over.

Store in an airtight container in the fridge for up to a week.

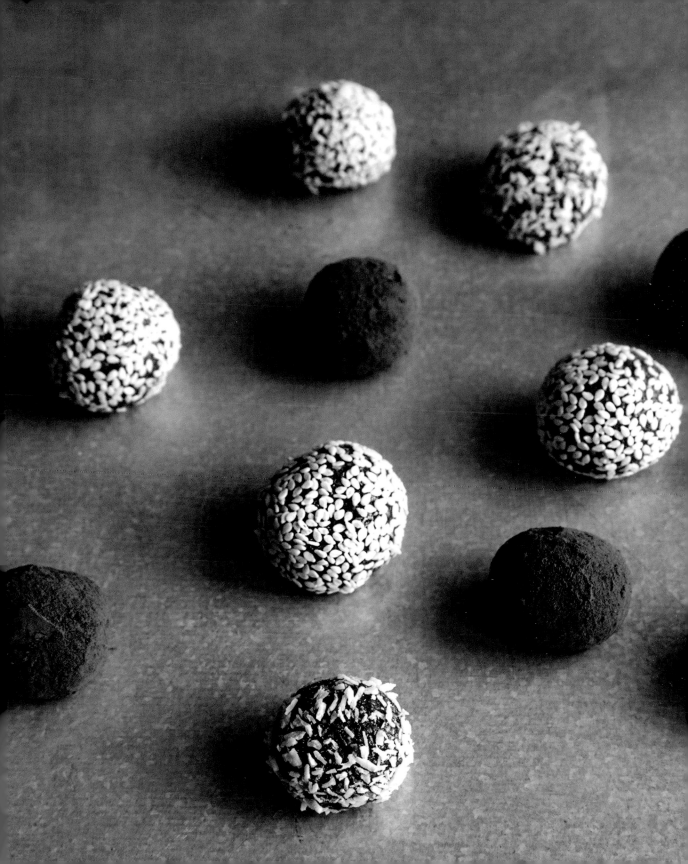

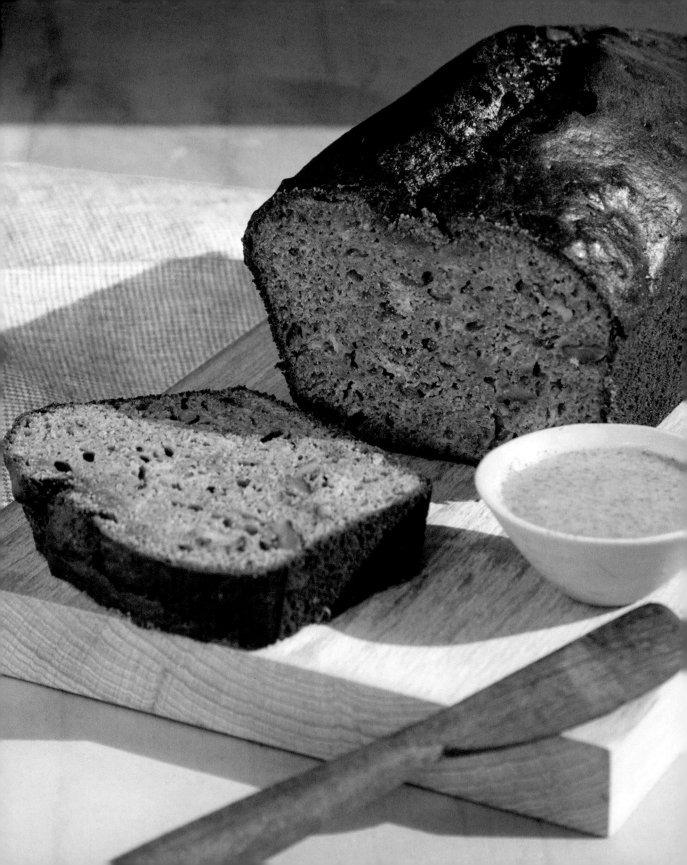

makes
1
loaf

You may have figured out by now that I eat a lot of bananas, but sometimes a few get over-ripe before I can use them all up. When that happens, I make this banana bread. I've pumped up the protein with chocolate protein powder and walnuts, which are also rich in omega-3s.

protein-packed banana bread

175g plain flour
100g coconut blossom sugar or
  light brown sugar
2 x 30g scoops of chocolate
  protein powder
2 teaspoons baking powder
2 eggs
4 tablespoons melted coconut oil
  or sunflower oil
4 tablespoons Greek yoghurt
4 medium-sized over-ripe bananas
  (about 500g unpeeled weight)
100g chopped walnuts
nut butter, to serve

Preheat the oven to 170°C. Line a 1lb loaf tin with a paper liner (you can buy these in the baking section of most supermarkets) or non-stick baking paper.

Put the flour, sugar, protein powder and baking powder in a bowl and stir together.

Crack the eggs into a jug, then add the oil and yoghurt and use a fork to whisk them together. Using the same fork, mash the bananas on a chopping board until they've broken down to a purée.

Pour the wet ingredients and the mashed bananas into the bowl with the dry ingredients and stir everything together with a wooden spoon or spatula until you have a smooth batter with no dry pockets of flour. Add the walnuts and give everything one last stir just to combine.

Transfer the batter to the lined loaf tin, then bake in the oven for 45 to 50 minutes, rotating the tin halfway through, until a skewer inserted into the middle of the bread comes out clean. If a little batter is clinging to the skewer, put the bread back in the oven for 5 more minutes and keep testing it at 5-minute intervals until it's done.

Transfer the tin to a wire rack and allow to cool for 10 minutes, then turn the bread out of the tin, peel off the paper and allow to cool completely on the rack before slicing and spreading with your favourite nut butter. Store any leftovers in an airtight container or wrapped tightly in foil in the fridge for three days, but I guarantee that it won't last that long!

treats

serves

2

This is just as good for breakfast as it is for dessert, in which case you could scatter some granola (page 162) on top instead of the hazelnuts. If you want to make this even more of a treat, make a quick and easy chocolate sauce by whisking a tiny splash of milk into a few spoonfuls of a high-protein chocolate spread until it's a thin enough consistency for drizzling and use this instead of the honey.

grilled pears with greek yoghurt & hazelnuts

2 large ripe pears
coconut oil cooking spray
4 tablespoons 0% fat
   high-protein vanilla Greek
   yoghurt
pinch of ground cinnamon
4 teaspoons roughly chopped
   hazelnuts
honey, for drizzling

Cut the pears in half lengthways and scoop out the core using a teaspoon or melon baller.

Set a chargrill pan over a high heat. When it's really hot, spritz the cut side of the pears with the coconut oil cooking spray, then place on the hot pan, cut side down. Grill for 3 minutes without moving them, until nice char marks form and the pears have softened a bit. Remove the pan from the heat.

Put the pears on your serving plates, grilled side up so that you can see the char marks. Add 1 tablespoon of yogurt on top of each pear half, scatter over a pinch of ground cinnamon, then top with 1 teaspoon of chopped hazelnuts.

Finish with a drizzle of honey over everything.

treats

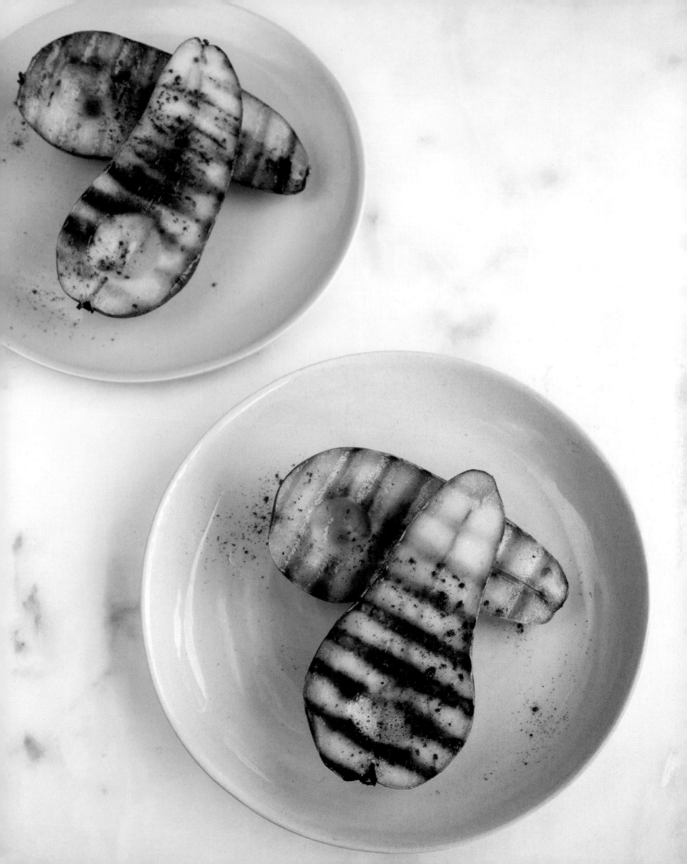

makes
15

You could give these a Nutella vibe by using finely chopped hazelnuts and hazelnut butter instead of the almonds and almond butter.

chocolate & almond energy bites

30g oats
30g finely chopped almonds
1 x 30g scoop of chocolate
  protein powder
3 tablespoons almond butter
2 tablespoons honey
4 teaspoons almond milk
pinch of salt
a small handful of goji berries
  (optional), to decorate

Put everything except the goji berries in a food processor or blender and blitz until it comes together into a ball. If you think it looks a bit dry, add another teaspoon of milk and blend again.

Line a small 17cm x 25cm baking tray with cling film, then transfer the mixture from the food processor to the lined tray. Using damp hands or the back of a spoon that you've run under the cold tap, press the mixture down firmly in an even layer that takes up only half the tray. Scatter over the goji berries (if using).

Put the tray in the freezer for at least 30 minutes, until the slab has set firm. Alternatively, you could follow the instructions for the protein balls on page 194 and roll them into balls instead.

Using the cling film, lift the slab out of the baking tray on to a chopping board. Using a sharp knife, cut into bite-sized pieces about 2.5cm square.

Store in an airtight container in the fridge for up to a week or a month in the freezer.

treats

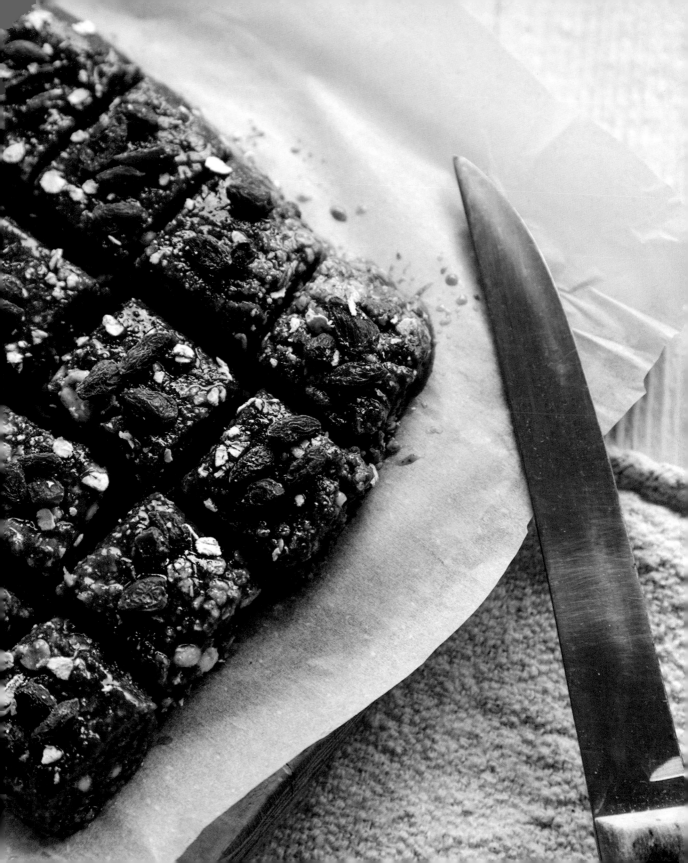

serves

4

This has all the creamy richness of ice cream but none of the guilt! In fact, it's so healthy that you could have it for breakfast – I sometimes put a scoop on top of my stuffed French toast (page 168).

I've kept things super simple with just two ingredients here, but you could add all sorts of extras to this, like a tablespoon of peanut butter, high-protein chocolate spread, maple syrup or honey, your favourite finely chopped nuts, or a pinch of ground cinnamon or nutmeg.

Frozen bananas will make your smoothies extra creamy too, so if you've got a bunch of bananas lying around that are on the verge of getting over-ripe, freeze them and store them in ziplock freezer bags, ready to throw into the blender or whip up into this dessert.

treats

two-ingredient banana ice cream

4 ripe bananas
1 x 30g scoop of protein powder
 (any flavour)
maple syrup or honey,
 for drizzling (optional)
cacao nibs, to serve (optional)

First line a large baking tray with non-stick baking paper. Peel the bananas and cut into slices, then put on the lined tray in a single layer. Pop into the freezer for at least 2 hours, until all the slices are frozen solid.

Put the frozen bananas and protein powder in a food processor or high-powered blender and blitz until creamy. This will take a few minutes, so don't worry when it looks crumbly at first or is spinning around your food processor as one big ball – just keep blending until it's a silky-smooth consistency. Serve immediately drizzled with some maple syrup or honey if you want a little extra sweetness and some cacao nibs scattered on top if liked.

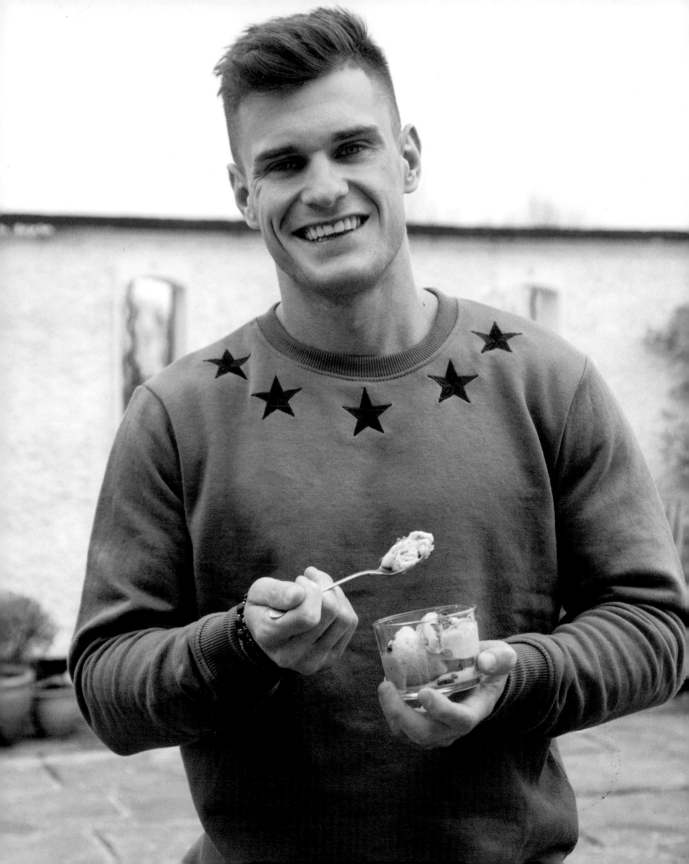

ACKNOWLEDGEMENTS

I want to give a big thanks to everyone who helped bring this book to life. In my short years of business and entrepreneurship I have quickly learned that you will not get very far on your own. Surround yourself with the right people and build that amazing team.

My family, especially my sister Rosalind. They are my real day ones and are the people who will always be honest with me. My mother is one of the toughest people I know and has taught me to never, ever give up no matter what happens. Roz has been one of my best mates since I can remember!

A big thanks to Susan McKeever. There are some days when even I'm not feeling it and Susan would always be there to sit down with me and help me get those words on the paper. We would also have a laugh while doing so which I think is extremely important! She made me realize how much of a bro I am and that most people wouldn't understand a single sentence of mine if I was to talk to them the way I talk to my gym buddies.

A huge shout out to Kristin Jensen for helping me concoct new and exciting recipes – no plain boiled chicken and rice here!

I'm honoured to be able to say that I had one of my oldest and dearest friends give me his valuable input on this book. Aaron O'Farrell is not only an amazing writer himself, but a comedian in my eyes too. If only our old principal could see us now.

A big thank you to my shoot team: Bríd O'Donovan, Niamh Browne, Barry Hirst and Clare Wilkinson. I will never forget the days we had down in the cottage having the chats, taking photos, cooking delicious food and, of course, eating it afterwards!

Thanks to my brilliant book designer, Nikki Dupin, for her creative energy and input.

To my editor, Claire Pelly, and to Michael McLoughlin at Penguin Random House Ireland. My life can be a little crazy and hectic at times (most of the time) and these are the two that kept me on my toes and honestly made it all happen. I can truly say I couldn't have done it without them: they are like my book parents! There were moments of stressful deadlines and reality checks but also moments in the office where we would be close to tears laughing! An amazing duo.

And most of all to the readers, the LF Army, from all the people who may just be joining the journey now to the people who have been with me since day one, the George the Cat days, making videos on that old couch and drinking poverty soda. Thanks for sticking with me, there is so much more to come.